100 SECRET BEAUTY RECIPES *of* THE FRENCH STARS

CAMILLE OBADIA

I would like to dedicate this book for my two wonderful children Assaf and Olivier, to my daughter-in-law Santa, to my two amazing grandchildren Dante and Niko who love to surf and skateboard and to my mother Rachel who always believed in me and who is very special to me.

About the Author:
The Story of Camille Obadia

Camille Obadia has over 50 years of experience in the beauty industry. After studying medical cosmetic care, post-surgery aesthetics, aromatherapy, phytotherapy and Essential oils for more than 10 years, Camille began her career at elite Paris clinics. She treated famous French movie stars and television actresses, royalty, models, artists, and top designers.

Camille has been a frequent consultant for, and is widely quoted in, national beauty magazines and newspapers, and on French television. As a skin care expert, she has published numerous articles in French magazines such as Vogue, Cosmopolitan, and Sante who have called upon her to share her expertise.

In 2004, Camille collaborated with French specialists and doctors to establish the *College European* De *Formation Continue Paramedical Esthetic* in Paris. The school's mission is to re-educate medical, paramedical, and aesthetic professionals.

With the French governmental alliance certification, operational logistics, curriculum development, recruitment of trains/ faculty and coordination of graduate placement.

After many years of experience, Camille decided to develop her own makeup and skin care line, collaborating with doctors, engineers and chemists to create products that protect against the effects of pollution, increase oxygenation, maintain collagen levels to keep the skin healthy and to fight the aging process.

For years, Camille had many American clients who would visit her Paris clinic. So, in 2010, she decided to open her first French beauty clinic in New York... "BEAUTE OBLIGE".

Her clinic became the secret of chic New Yorkers, fashion and beauty editors, designers, supermodels, and celebrities like Sofia Vergara

Camille's extensive experience and knowledge in the beauty industry led her to create her own beauty guide. It is filled with valuable and easy to understand information, with a comprehensive list of natural, organic face and body products and self-care guidance. She provides tools to empower you to take control of your own beauty routine at home.

Although there are many beauty books on the market, Camille was inspired to write this book to provide accessible and helpful methods for men and women to take care of themselves at home and further the success of professional treatments.

Disclaimer:

Doctor Lionnel Michat

cardiologist, phytotherapy and aromatherapy specialist.

_____

Against all odds, Camille Obadia, a beauty specialist, and I, a cardiologist working in heart transplants, crossed paths. Throughout our countless meetings, both of us had to remain very open-minded.

As a specialist in a highly technical environment, I couldn't have been further from the world of cosmetics and beauty, yet the limits of certain therapeutics in my field led me to turn to natural therapeutics and essential oils, and to open up new approaches.

Meanwhile, Camille Obadia, as a specialist in the use of products to enhance women's beauty, slow down their aging process and to fight wrinkles, quickly understood the interest of natural products and essential oils. Camille Obadia took advantage of her experience to create new product lines with surprising results. Today she has a range of natural, ecological and organic products that she can offer to French stars.

It is around the creation of these products that we met, when she asked me to teach at her European college paramedical

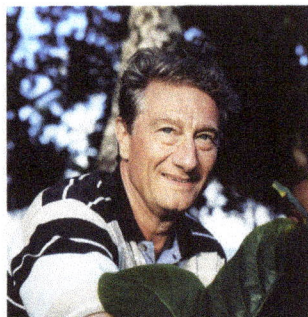

aesthetic in Paris, France. We were thus able to benefit from each other's knowledge and experience to be able to use natural products, plants and essential oils in both of our fields, because these plants have multiple virtues that can be used in therapeutics but also in cosmetics.

In her book, Camille Obadia, inspired by her years spent with French stars, demonstrates a range of beauty products, giving you the compositions allowing you to make your own beauty products at home. We can congratulate and thank her for her great work in helping women feel beautiful.

Contents

CHAPTER 1

The Skin, Its Needs, Its Functions

The skin is a sensitive and deeply superficial organ.

Skin color is classified in shades of white, brown and black.

Women tend to have a lighter complexion; they produce less melanin than men.

Genetics and hormones play an important role in defining the color of the complexion.

The skin evolves as we age. Fat cells shrink and the skin loses its elasticity. The most common inconvenience is the premature appearance of wrinkles.

THE SKIN'S FUNCTIONS:

- Thermoregulatory protection.
- Absorption.
- Immune protection.
- Preservation of the hydrolipidic film of its different layers.
- Preservation of the skin's moisture.
- Permeability.
- Maintenance of a homogeneous and thermal skin temperature.
- Preservation of skin texture.

PHYSIOLOGICAL SIGNS OF SKIN AGING:

- A decrease in secretions.
- Dryness.
- Increased skin irritation.
- Loss of skin elasticity.
- Decrease in blood fluid.
- Decrease in collagen production and loss of elasticity.
- Poor healing.
- Hyperpigmentation of the skin.

THE SKIN AND ITS NEEDS

- Water is vital to preserve young and radiant skin.
- 70% of the human body is made of water.
- Water is vital for the skin and body's health, as well as its youthfulness.

THE SKIN'S LAYERS:

THE EPIDERMIS:

- The epidermis is the outer layer.
- It protects us from various toxins and bacteria.
- It preserves the moisture and lipid content of our skin.
- It prevents the weakening of the skin.

THE DERMIS:

- The dermis is an elastic support tissue.
- The dermis contains hyaluronic acid, elastin and collagen.
- The dermis contains the vascular network.

THE HYPODERMIS:

- Protects and slows skin aging.
- Protects the skin's thermal and energetic effect.
- Ensures good mechanical functioning of the skin.

THE DIFFERENT TYPES OF SKIN:

- Dry skin: is often thin, dry and has a dull complexion.
- Oily skin: has a shiny appearance, prone to acne.
- Mixed skin: the centre of the face is greasy (shiny).

BROWN SPOTS:

- Brown spots are mainly caused by prolonged exposure to ultraviolet rays.
- Melanin is concentrated in certain areas of skin and brown spots appear: this phenomenon can happen in both young and older skins.
- Hormonal and contraceptive pills may also cause brown spots in contexts of prolonged sun exposure.

SKIN AGING AND BROWN SPOTS:

- Age spots are usually common starting the age of 40.
- Sun and UV exposure trigger melanin overproduction.
- Age spots may be present on the hands, face, neck and cleavage.
- A thorough solar protection relies on the choice of sun-blocking products.

MEN'S SKIN:

- By nature, men's skin is more resistant than that of the woman.
- The epidermis cells are more numerous, as well as firmer, since their skin is reinforced with collagen for hormonal reasons.
- Usually sagging skin appears later in men than in women.
- The production of sebum is greater in men, due to the higher rate of testosterone levels, equivalent to 10 times that of a woman: this causes a greater stimulation of the sebaceous glands, promoting an oilier skin.
- The blood flow is more abundant, more conducive to aggravated redness by shaving.
- The texture of men's skin is more absorbent when it comes to serums and creams. After shaving, the skin is dry and irritated, it is necessary to moisturize it with a soothing after-shave balm.
- It is also recommended to gently cleanse the skin to help the skin better absorb the balm and cream.

ITCHY SKIN (INFLAMMATION OF DRY SKIN):

- Itchy skin usually manifests itself with an unpleasant urge to scratch oneself.
- Itchy skin can happen on the face, neck, chest area as well as the rest of the body.
- The skin presents redness with a rough aspect and small bumps appear at the surface. These are unpleasant signs of dry skin.
- The cold, frequent use of heating and air-conditioning, as well as baths and hot temperatures can cause dry skin.
- The skin may react and can be allergic to certain medications.
- The skin may react to hormonal imbalance or kidney failure.
- The skin may react to soaps and body lotions that are too fragrant.
- The skin may react to excessive stress and perspiration.

STEP 1:

- Schedule an appointment with a dermatologist immediately, in order to obtain an allergy test.

STEP 2:

- Spray the affected parts of the skin with thermal water.
- Moisturize the skin regularly, several times a day with emollients.
- In the shower, make sure you use soap-less body wash, dry your skin immediately and moisturize with a moisturizer rich in vitamin A.

REDNESS, FACIAL FLUSHING, ERYTHEMA, COUPROSE AND ROSACEA

FACIAL FLUSHING

- Fragile skin types tend to present redness. With time, redness can become recurrent and, eventually, permanent.
- Such degrees of redness are called: FACIAL FLUSHING—It is a temporary redness that may disappears in a few minutes.

ERYTHEMA

- A condition where redness is local, persistent and permanent, with red patches on the cheeks.

COUPEROSE:

- An aggravation of erythema inducing the appearance of small red vessels on the cheeks and often on the chin.

5

ROSACEA:

- Condition where small, red pimples appear, revealing a chronic skin infection. Often located on the nose, cheeks, forehead, chin and chest area.
- Fair skins are more prone to rosacea, especially following the consumption of alcohol.
- Avoid unprotected sun exposure.
- Avoid overly spicy foods, hot drinks, and alcoholic beverages.

DID YOU KNOW:

- Creams and other external skin care products do not reach the deep layers of the skin. Instead, cosmetic nutrients help to nourish the dermis via the action of micro-nutrients on the deeper layers, where the skin's aging process stems from.
- An accurate dosage of cosmetic nutrients is essential

THE CEBACEOUS GLANDS:

- The role of the sebaceous glands is to balance the hydrolipidic film of the skin.
- To balance the sebum production of each part of the skin, (forehead, cheeks, nose and chin).

PERSPIRATION:

- The role of perspiration is to balance the smell of the skin. to distribute perspiration to the whole skin.
- To balance and feed the skin with oxygen.

COSMETIC AGENTS THAT MAY SLOW DOWN THE SKIN'S AGING PROCESS

LOTIONS:

- intended to clean, depollute the skin and ensure a soft, protective make-up removal with the aim of preserving the skin's levels of Retinol, AHA, vitamins E, C, Q10, and trace elements.

CREAMS:

- An important contribution to our skin, they bring vitamins and antioxidants to our skin.
- Oil soaps protect the PH of our skin and balance its hydration.

THE SKIN AND THE SUN:

TANNED SKIN AND SUNBURN:

- A tanned skin ages more quickly following an intense and long exposure to the sun.
- Ultraviolet rays cause 1st and 2nd degree burn to the skin.
- Repeated sunburns can cause skin cancer and the appearance of brown spots.
- It is imperative to use a sunscreen adapted to your skin
- Eat fruits and vegetables containing beta carotene (vitamin A), drink enough water per day.
- Use a body milk or lotion after sun exposure, immediately after your shower.
- Be sure to apply sunscreen before, during and after going in the water.
- Cover your head and face with a large straw hat.
- Use aloe vera gel or tamanu oil to soothe a sunburn
- Apply cold compresses to relieve a sunburn.

DIFFERENCES BETWEEN UVA AND UVB RAYS:

- UV rays are the ultraviolet radiation emitted by the sun, the 2 types:
- UVA
- UVB
- UVA and UVB rays reach the surface of the Earth.
- UVB rays are responsible for sunburns.

THE EFFECTS OF UVA RAYS:

- They are less visible but no less harmful.
- They penetrate deep into the dermis.
- WHAT IS SPF:
- The sun protection factor. It is therefore the level of UV sun protection.

WHAT DOES A 'WET SKIN' LABEL MEAN?

- This product can be applied on wet skin.
- The formula contains ingredients that protect the epidermis.
- Its level of protection is long lasting.

WHAT DOES PHOTOSTABLE MEAN:

- This statement explains that the product does not lose its effectiveness during sun exposure and prevents UV rays from penetrating the skin.

INFRA-RED LIGHT: SHOULD THEY BE AVOIDED

- Infra-red rays penetrate the hypodermis.
- They lead to the production of free radicals, damage the cells, contribute to the loss of skin firmness and accelerate the appearance of wrinkles.

NAILS:

- Nails are composed of keratinized cells with uninterrupted growth.

INFORMATION ON SUNSCREENS: CHEMICAL AND MINERAL SUNSCREENS:

There are 2 types of sunscreens that protect the skin from the sun:

1. CHEMICAL:

- Chemical sunscreens are formulated in laboratories.
- They provide UV protection.
- It protects the skin from the inside to the outside.
- Some skins do not tolerate chemical sunscreens.

2. MINERAL SUNSCREENS

- These sunscreens are manufactured with mineral powders:
- Zinc oxide.
- Titanium dioxide.
- These ingredients remain on the surface of the skin.
- They act on the skin as a barrier, they prevent UVA and UVB rays to penetrate the skin.

CHAPTER 2

Face Peels

THE HISTORY OF PEELS:

- Face peels have been around for a long time.

- In ancient times, women exfoliated their skin with citric acid (lemon juice), or with a decoction of sugar cane.

- At the beginning of the 20th century, scientific peels appeared and were supervised by the medical profession.

- In general, peels are used to reduce skin issues.

- Peels may help in dealing with dull skin, slow down the process of aging, giving the skin radiance, softness and youth.

AESTHETIC PEELS:

The word peeling is equivalent to "stimulation".

Usually peels performed in institutes are peels based on 0% to 30% glycolic acid in concentration.

These peels do not treat dark spots. These peels carried out in a salon stimulate the epidermis to the dermis.

- Peels performed in institutes may help to tighten pores, fade brown spots, and reduce the depth of fine lines.
- It allows to obtain a cleared complexion, as well as an immediate radiance effect.
- The beautician may suggest peels every 15 days in a beauty salon for a period of 6 weeks in order to obtain satisfactory results.
- Cosmetic peels are usually achievable on all kinds of skins, including fair skin and dark skin.

MEDICAL PEELS:

THE COSMO PEEL:

It is a peel which is performed by a doctor. It boosts the skin and evens out fine lines. This peel is usually performed 3 times a year.

THE SPOT PEEL:

This peel is usually suitable for all kinds of skin.

It is effective on pigmentation spots and it must be performed by a cosmetic doctor or dermatologist.

DEEP PEEL:

- This peel must be performed by the doctor.
- The goal of this peel is to obtain a rejuvenation of 7 to 10 years.
- (It all depends on the age of the patient).
- The skin is then lifted, the wrinkles disappear, thanks to the new elastic synthetic fibers and collagen.
- The final results appear after 5 to 6 months.

THE DISADVANTAGES OF A DEEP PEEL:

It is a painful peel, because of the intense peeling of the skin it induces. You must plan to stay at home and rest for 56 days following the treatment.

The skin color will remain pink for a few days, then lighten.
    If you have deep scars, you might need to repeat this peel after 7 months.

WHAT IS A TCA PEELING?

ᔄ It is a very superficial peel recommended for oily and dilated pores, as well as for skin with dark spots.

ᔄ This peel is performed only by the doctor.

OTHER SPECIFIC TREATMENTS PERFORMED BY A DOCTOR ONLY:

ᔄ LASER!

ᔄ PULSED LIGHT!

ᔄ IPL.

Usually, these treatments give immediate results.

THE RETINOL:

ᔄ The role of Retinol is to stimulate the skin's elastin.

ᔄ Reduces brown spots.

ᔄ It is concentrated in vitamin A which may help the degradation and regulation of melanin responsible for brown spots.

ᔄ It is usually recommended to use it as a beauty treatment every other day at bedtime.

ᔄ Retinol acts on both the dermis and the epidermis.

ᔄ It stimulates cell renewal and promotes skin radiance.

ᔄ Retinol applied topically to the skin improves and balances the pores.

ᔄ It acts on the skin on the surface and in depth.

In conclusion:
    RETINOL is a form of vitamin A contained in cosmetic formulas such as Retinol Acetate and Retinyl Palmitate.

ON THE SURFACE

It has an exfoliating effect and smooths the texture of the skin, making it more radiant and reducing brown spots.

IN DEPTH:

It stimulates the production of collagen and elastin and increases the concentration of hyaluronic acid for a beneficial effect on the skin. The concentration of Retinol is usually less than 0.3%.

PRECAUTIONS:

Never use Retinol on already irritated skin. Do not simultaneously use products containing glycolic acid.

- Avoid contact with eyes.
- Avoid any sun exposure without a high protection sunscreen.

GLYCOLIC ACID:

- Glycolic acid is a fruit acid obtained from sugar cane, beets or grapes.
- It is a small molecule of fruit acids which is easily absorbed by the skin and stimulates cellular activity.
- GLYCOLIC ACID HAS AN EFFECT ON: the elimination of dead cells from the surface of the skin the hydration of the stratum corneum. the reparation of melanin cells, unification and brightening of the complexion. the production of collagen and elastin, providing a firming and toning effect.
- Glycolic acid integrated in cosmetic creams and peels improves the texture of the skin, provides the skin with better hydration.

OXYGENATION:

It can usually be used on all types of skin.

The concentration of glycolic acid in cosmetic creams is usually concentrated from 4% to 15%.

ON OILY SKIN:

- It is used as a regulator of seborrhea.

ON MATURE AND DRY SKIN:

- It is an excellent anti-wrinkle and brightening product.
  Creams can be applied in the evening to clean, dry skin 1 to 3 times / week.

SPECIFIC TREATMENTS WHICH ARE PERFORMED BY DERMATOLOGISTS:

- lasers. intense pulsed light.
- IPL
- Usually, these specific treatments give immediate and satisfactory results.

ORGANIC SILICON ON THE SKIN:

Organic silicon is a powerful and essential trace element which binds to large collagen molecules in the dermis to ensure its structure. It is essential for good hydration and suppleness of the skin. Silicon stimulates the formation of collagen fibers and firm tissue skin.

CHAPTER 3

Nutrition of the Skin

THE SYNERGIE OF NUTRITION ON THE SKIN:

- The modification of metabolism of the aging cells slows the reproduction of collagen and provokes the degradation of elastin.

- Smoking, alcohol, being exposed, the cold and pollution affect the hormonal imbalance.

- For all of these reasons, the hormonal functioning is slowed, and the aging of skin is premature.

- The research on nutrition have made it possible to define the relations between the skin and nutrition as well as the nutritional conditions necessary for a good maintenance of the quality of the skin.

- The vitamins, oligos elements and antioxidants may help against wrinkles.

COSMETIC NUTRIENTS, DIETARY SUPPLEMENTS AND OUR SKIN:

- Cosmetic nutrients and dietary supplements target the care of hair, nails and may help in the fight of age.

- The cosmetic nutrients will act by bringing the micro-nutrients, vitamins, antioxidants, collagen, hyaluronic acid, capable of slowing down the loss of elasticity and the hydration of the skin.
- Nutrients are cosmetics which may slow down the process of aging and acts as a preventive barrier.

DIETARY SUPPLEMENTS AND THE SKIN:

- They act from the inside to the outside.
- They are complementary to the creams and serums that we use daily.
- They exist in the form of capsules, pills, drinks and infusions.
- They may help in the fight against aging.
- Reinforces the defense of the skin.
- Some may have a concentrated supply of vitamin C, E, zinc lycopene and magnesium.

HOW TO CHOOSE YOUR COSMETIC NUTRIENTS FOR THE SKIN:

- The antique oxidant: resveratrol.
- Hyaluronic acid.
- Saturated fatty acids (Omega 3+6).
- Anti oxidants (vitamins C, E and zinc).
- Rosmarinus acid which acts on the firmness of the skin.

MINERAL WATERS:

The benefits of mineral and sparkling waters on our skin: soda water, is rich in magnesium.

CALCIUM

The concentration of calcium in the diet is more beneficial for our skin than calcium as a dietary supplement.

ANTIOXIDANTS AND THEIR BENEFITS ON OUR SKIN:

- They may reduce inflammation of the skin cells.
- Smooth out wrinkles.
- They may help the cutaneous aging, slow down the appearance of wrinkles, protect our skin from pollution, accelerate cell production thanks to the awakening of elastin.
- May contribute to the regeneration of collagen and vitamin E.
- May protects the fibroblasts, contributes to the vital contribution in tonicity and hydration of the skin.

WE FIND THEM IN:

- St. John's Wort oil, muscat rose oil, organic vegetable oils, in red fruit acids, goji berries, guava and pomegranate.

TRACE ELEMENTS AND THEIR BENEFITS FOR OUR SKIN:

5 ACTIVE TRACE ELEMENTS AND THEIR BENEFITS ON THE SKIN: COPPER, MANGANESE, SELENIUM, SILICON, ZINC.

SELENIUM:

- Selenium has an anti-oxidizing role, it decreases the general oxidative stress, protects the cells and repairs the damage of the skin due to solar rays.

COPPER:

- It is a trace element essential for the skin.
- It preserves the skin's collagen level.

MANGANESE:

- Has a major role in the protection of the skin and preserves collagen.

ZINC:

- It preserves the proteins and collagen of the skin.
- It is an ideal anti-inflammatory for oily and acne-prone skin.

SILICON:

- Silicon is a powerful and essential trace element that binds to the large molecules of the dermis to ensure its structure.
- It stimulates the production of collagen.
- It stimulates the formation of collagen fibers, maintains the hydration and tone of the skin.

GLYCOLIC ACID HOW IT ACTS ON OUR SKIN:

- Glycolic acid is a fruit acid obtained from sugar cane, beet or grapes.
- It is a small fruit acid molecule that allows a very good absorption in the skin and stimulates cell activity.
- It acts as an exfoliant and removes dead cells from the surface of the skin.
- It acts as a powerful moisturizer of the stratum corneum.
- It unify and brighten the complexion.

↶ It participates in the reproduction of collagen and elastin; it reaffirms and tones the skin.

↶ Glycolic acid is integrated in creams and face masks.

COSMETICS:

↶ It improves the texture of the skin and brings to the skin a better hydration and oxygenation.

↶ Glycolic acid can be used on all skin types: young, mature, oily and normal skin.

↶ The concentration of glycolic acid in cosmetic creams is usually concentrated from 4% to 15%.

↶ ON OILY SKINS, glycolic acid acts:

↶ As a regulator of seborrhea.

↶ ON MATURE AND DRY SKINS, it is excellent for brightening and may help prevent wrinkles.

↶ Glycolic acid-based creams are applied in the evening to clean and dry skin 1-3 times a week.

VITAMINS AND THEIR EFFECTS ON OUR SKIN:

VITAMIN A (RETINOL OR BETA CAROTENE):

↶ Vitamin A has anti-oxidizing virtues with an important contribution of collagen to the skin.

↶ Vitamin A activates cell renewal and hydrates the skin.

VITAMIN B2, (RIBOFLAVIN):

↶ Contributes to the tonicity and flexibility of the skin.

↶ IT IS CONCENTRATED IN: Green vegetables, camembert and yoghurt.

VITAMIN B3, (NIACIN, NICOTINIC ACID):

- Its role is to regenerate and hydrate the skin in depth.
- It activates the production of collagen.

- IT CAN BE FOUND IN: Fish, poultry, mushrooms, brewer's yeast, hazelnuts, peanuts and brown rice.

VITAMIN B5, (PANTOTHENIC ACID):

- This vitamin contributes to the skin to be smooth and soft.

- IT CAN BE FOUND IN: Sweet potatoes, milk, lentils, oats, pumpkin and cashews.

VITAMIN B1, (THIAMINE):

- This vitamin helps with carbohydrates and energy for the balance of the skin.

- IT CAN BE FOUND IN: Dry vegetables, brewer's yeast, beef liver, fish, green beans and eggs.

VITAMIN B6, (PYRIDOXINE):

- This vitamin helps to store proteins and carbohydrates.

- IT CAN BE FOUND IN: Brewer's yeast, avocado, lentils, banana, sunflower seeds and eggs.

VITAMIN C, (SCORBUTIC ACID):

- This vitamin participates in the radiance of the skin.
- It evens out the skin.
- Preserves the youthfulness of the skin.
- It fights the signs of age and may reduces the appearance of wrinkles.

- It helps to preserve the elasticity of the skin against stretch marks.
- IT CAN BE FOUND IN: Mushrooms, vegetables, fish liver oil, milk, butter, cheese, liver, chicken and sardines.

VITAMIN E (TOCOPHEROL):

- Vitamin E is essential when it comes to cell protection within the skin.
- Vitamin E helps to stimulate the production of collagen and protein, restoring the skin's elasticity.
- It evens out and softens the skin.
- It moisturizes fine and sensitive skin and may calm skin irritations.
- IT IS FOUND IN: Cereal, olives, egg yolk, avocado, butter, sardines, hazelnuts, almonds and organic vegetable oils.

VITAMIN K (PHYTONADIONE, TOCOPHEROL):

- Vitamin K helps to soothe red and itchy skin.
- It revitalizes and restores the skin's radiance and healthy appearance.
- IT IS FOUND IN: Dark chocolate, fresh ginger, sunflower seeds, garlic and fresh salmon.

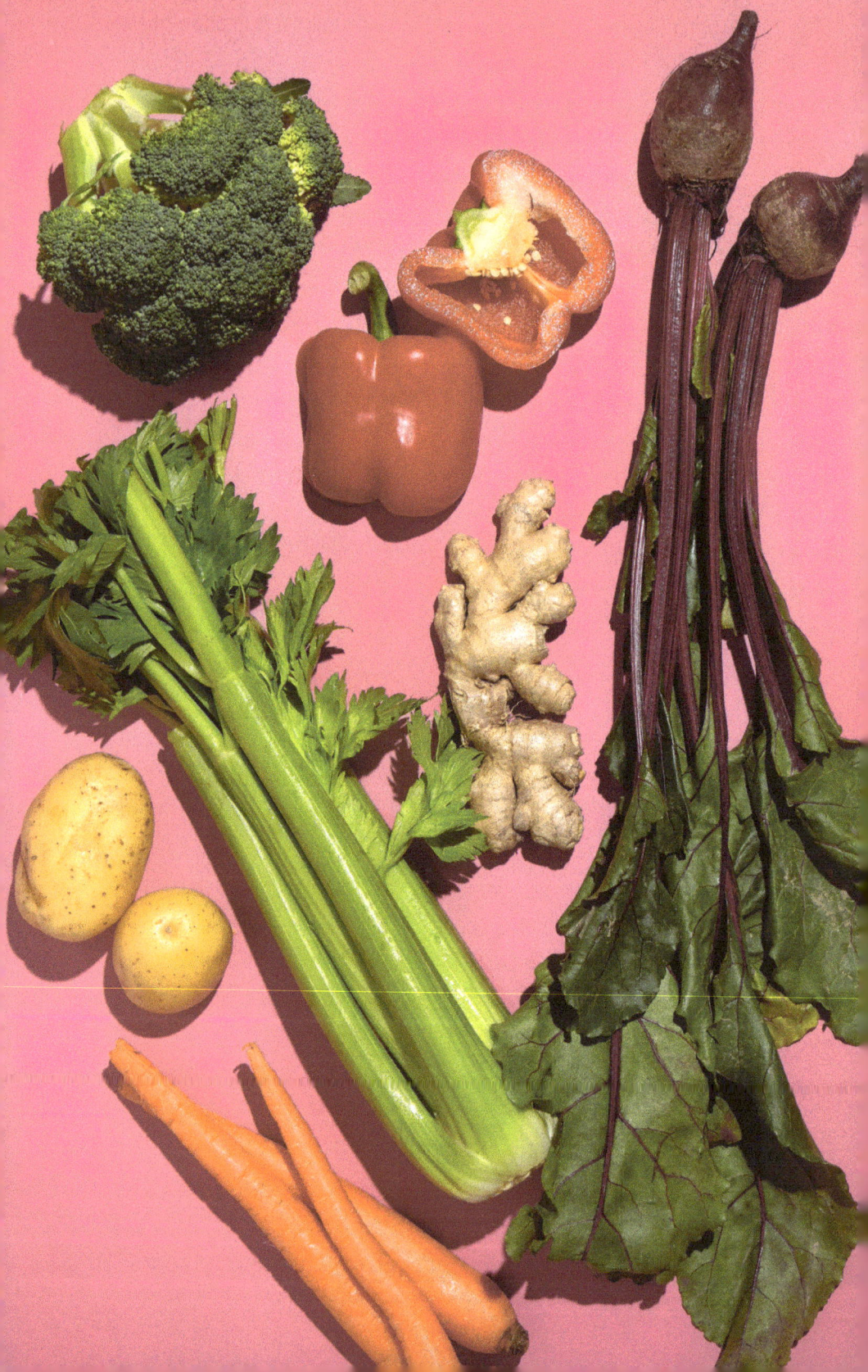

FRUITS AND VEGETABLES, THEIR BENEFITS FOR THE SKIN:

CARROT:

- It contains a high concentration of calcium, which is beneficial to the skin.
- It contains a high concentration of antioxidants.
- It balances and improves skin texture.

CUCUMBER:

- The cucumber is a very popular, depurative and diuretic vegetable
- It is rich in water (up to 90%), and in fiber.
- It is rich in vitamins A, B, C, E, and K.

POTATO:

- Rich in fiber, potassium, minerals, vitamins C, B1 B3, B5, magnesium and phosphorus.
- Concentrated in lysine, amino acids, proteins and lipids.
- Important source of iron, zinc, copper, magnesium and lutein.

RED BELL PEPPER:

- Rich in vitamins C and A, iron, sodium and potassium.
- Rich in fiber, giving it invigorating and antiseptic qualities.

BEET:

- Contains vitamins B, B9, A and C.
- Rich in carbohydrates and minerals

- Concentrated in folic acid, beta carotene, iron and sodium, magnesium and copper.

FRESH GINGER:

- Full of antioxidants.
- Rich in vitamins C, E, A, B1, B2, B3, B5, B6.

CELERY:

- Anti-aging food, rich in antioxidants, lutein, and beta carotene.
- Rich in vitamin A, trace elements, potassium, sodium, phosphorus, magnesium, iron, zinc,

- Contains soluble fibers and is rich in iron.
- Rich in enzymes, antioxidizing.

- Rich in trace elements, salts, vitamins and minerals.

manganese, selenium and a low-calorie food.
- Rich in fiber, calcium, iron, beta carotene, rich in carbohydrates, rich in protein, low-calorie.

OKRA:

- A powerful antioxidant, rich in vitamins A and C, may help against wrinkles.

- Rich in protein, calcium, iron and zinc.
- Rich in a soluble fiber.
- Rich in vitamin K12.

CILANTRO

- Rich in oxidants, concentrated in vitamin K, stimulates general tonus.

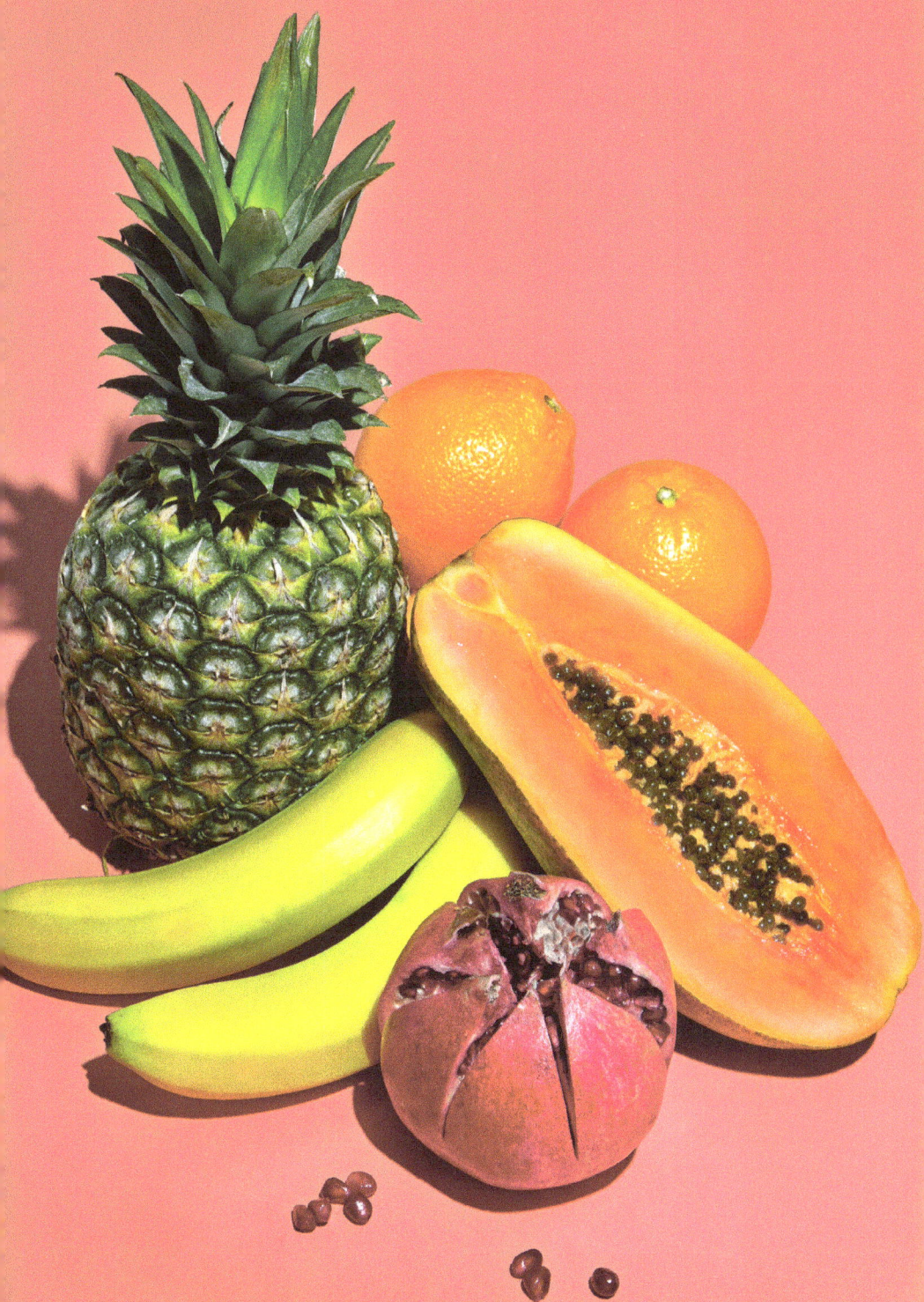

THE BENEFITS OF FRUIT ON OUR SKIN:

GRAPEFRUIT:

༄ Drains our body overall.

APPLE:

༄ It has a detoxifying action.

THE BENEFITS OF DRIED FRUITS:

PISTACHIOS:

༄ It is rich in vitamins: B6, K, B1.

༄ It is rich in fibres, helps with thinness.

༄ It is rich in antioxidants, copper, phosphorus and fibers.

༄ It is concentrated in manganese, rich in magnesium, potassium, vitamin E, protein and carbohydrates.

THE BENEFITS OF RED FRUITS:

༄ Red fruits contain a high concentration of natural pigments.

༄ They contain a high concentration of vitamin P, they are rich in antioxidants.

༄ Red fruits are rich in water.

SPICES AND THEIR BENEFITS FOR THE SKIN:

CINNAMON AND ITS VIRTUES:

༄ It is rich in antioxidants.

༄ It balances sebum on the skin.

SAFFRON:

- Rich in magnesium, source of vitamin B.
- Rich in beta carotene.

ROSEMARY:

- It is rich in anti oxidants, neutralizes free radicals linked to skin aging.

LAVENDER:

- Rich in acids.
- Can help preserves skin sagging.

PEPPER:

- It is a powerful anti oxidizer.

CHAPTER 4

Cosmetic Vegetable Oils and Their Benefits to the Skin

WHAT IS A VEGETABLE OIL?

A vegetable oil is a fatty substance extracted from a plant whose seeds, nuts or fruits are concentrated in lipids, rich in omega 6 and 9, as well as vitamins.

Vegetable oils have been used for many centuries for their properties, aromatherapies and benefits.

THEIR PROPERTIES AND THEIR INDICATIONS:

- The use of vegetable oils in the cosmetic industry is often associated with that of essential oils.
- Vegetable oils are rich in vitamins and omega 6 and 9.

COMPOSITION OF A VEGETABLE OIL:

- A vegetable oil contains 3 different kinds of fatty acids:
- Saturated acids.
- Polyunsaturated acids.
- Unsaturated acids.

- In the cosmetics industry, vegetable oils are regularly incorporated in the formulas of body milks, face creams and masks.
- Vegetable oils are often used with essential oils

SOME BENEFITS OF VEGETABLE OILS:

- Jojoba, shea and wheat germ oils are nourishing, anti-aging and rich in vitamin E.
- Deodorized coconut oil is regenerating, rich in vitamins and antioxidant.
- Olive and evening primrose oils are regenerating and anti-aging.
- Rice oil protects the skin.
- Most vegetable oils are rich in vitamins: F, A, Omega 3 and 6.
- Almond oil: hydrates, soothes and softens the skin; it is rich in vitamin A, E and K. is rich in uric acid and fights the appearance of stretch marks.
- Avocado oil is a powerful moisturizer on the skin.
- Carrot oil is rich in vitamins.
- Calendula oil has multiple soothing virtues.
- Grape seed oil is restructuring and restorative for the skin.
- Borage oil is revitalizing, protective and may help prevent stretch marks.
- Argan oil is rich in vitamin E and an antioxidant
- Jojoba oil comes from jojoba seeds. It moisturizes while revitalizing the Oil on the skin.
- Avocado oil is rich in vitamins A, B, C, D, E, H, K and PP. It may prevent stretch marks, softens and hydrates the skin.
- Nigella vegetable oil comes from the plant Nigella Sativa. It may prevent eczema and acne, is rich in fatty acid and is an antioxidant.
- Rosehip oil: it is rich in vitamins A, E, omega 3 and 6, protects and moisturizes the skin, suitable for dry and Irritated skin.

- Calendula oil may help calm sun burns.
- Carrot oil: it is rich in vitamins A and beta carotene.
- It promotes skin radiance.
- Borage oil is rich in vitamins A, D, E and K. It regenerates the skin, and preserves collagen fibers.
- Hemp oil: it is rich in omega 3 and 6, strengthens and moisturizes the skin.
- Wheat germ oil deeply hydrates the skin.
- Vegetable macadamia oil nourishes and hydrates the skin in depth, may prevent stretch marks. It is ideal for dehydrated and fragile skin.
- Hazelnut oil is ideal for combating the appearance of blackheads on the skin.
- Olive oil: Is healing, rich in omega 9, rich in polyphenols, rich in vitamins: A, E, D and K.
- Grape seed oil: it is rich in antioxidants, and anti-aging.
- Rosehip oil: is an antioxidant, is recommended for dry and dehydrated skin.
- Sesame oil: is recommended for performing body massages. It is concentrated in vitamin E, rich in lecithin, magnesium, and phosphorus.
- Caliphyllid inophyllum oil, called "tamanu oil". This wonderful oil is extracted from the nuts of a small tree native to Madagascar, East Africa and Australia. This oil is rich in omega 6 and 9, is concentrated in polyphenols, as well as rich in vitamin E. This oil calms the skin. Excellent skin moisturizer for dry and dehydrated skin.

HOW TO STORE VEGETABLE OILS:

In general, vegetable oils should be stored away from light and heat.

LIST OF VEGETABLE OILS: (ORGANIC IS PREFERRABLE)

- Sweet almond oil
- coconut oil
- avocado oil
- Nigella oil
- carrot oil
- rosehip oil
- tamanu oil
- castor oil
- grapefruit seed oil
- raspberry seed oil
- calendula oil
- grape seed oil
- borage oil
- argan oil
- hemp oil
- apricot
- macadamia oil
- walnut oil
- rosemary macerate oil
- sesame oil
- raspberry macerate oil
- evening primrose oil
- St. John's wort oil
- virgin olive oil
- jojoba oil.

EXAMPLE OF A PREPARATION OF YOUR BODY MASSAGE OIL:

- Usually, all organic vegetable oils can be used in your body massage oil formulas.

EXAMPLE:

- 1 glass 50ml glass bottle, not transparent.
- 50 ml of vegetable oil.
- 5 drops of essential oil of your choice, (you can use 2 kinds)

HOW TO SUCCEED IN THE CREATION OF A RELAXATION OIL:

It is recommended to use organic vegetable oils: organic sweet almond oil, organic sunflower oil, virgin and organic olive oil, organic jojoba oil, macadamia oil, organic coconut oil, evening primrose oil.

SOME BENEFITS OF VEGETABLE OILS:

- Jojoba, Shea, and wheat germ oils are nourishing and rich in vitamin E, as well as anti-aging.
- Coconut oil sublimates the skin.
- Vegetable oils (such as olive oil and evening primrose) are regenerating and anti-aging.
- Rice oil protects the skin and is anti-aging.
- All these oils are rich in vitamins: F, A, Omega 3 and 6.
- These oils are restorative.

LIST OF VEGETABLE OILS:

Used for many centuries for their properties, their aromatherapy and their benefits: rich in vitamins, can be used in beauty cream formulas and body oil milks.

- Sweet almond vegetable oil (hydrates, soothes and softens the skin, rich in vitamin A and E.
- Coconut vegetable oil, deodorized, regenerating, rich in vitamins: A and E, antioxidant, renews skin cells, rich in vitamin K, may help reduce dark circles, may help prevent stretch marks.
- Organic avocado vegetable oil, powerful moisturizer on the skin.
- Nigella vegetable oil
- Carrot vegetable oil, rich in vitamins.
- Hazelnut oil.
- Rosehip oil.
- Tamanu (caliphyllid inophyllum) oil.
- Castor oil.
- Grapefruit seed oil
- Raspberry seed oil
- Calendula oil: soothing.
- Grape seed oil: restructuring, restorative.

- Borage oil: revitalizing, protective, anti-stretch marks.
- Argan oil: antioxidant, rich in vitamin E.
- Hemp vegetable oil
- Apricot kernel oil
- Macadamia oil
- Vegetable oil from macerated rosemary.
- Organic sesame oil.
- Vegetable oil from macerated raspberries.
- Evening primrose oil.
- St. John's Wort oil.
- Organic Nigella Oil.
- Organic virgin olive oil.
- Jojoba oil: this oil comes from the seeds of the jojoba tree, moisturizes the skin, revitalizes the skin and anti-aging.

CHAPTER 5

Essential Oils and Their Use On The Skin

PRECAUTIONS TO BE TAKEN IN THE USE OF ESSENTIAL OILS

- Avoid the eyes.
- Keep essential oils out of the reach of children.
- Do not use essential oils if you are pregnant.
- Not for babies.
- Avoid the use of essential oils on irritated skin.
- Essential oils are prohibited for people at medical risk.

Essential oils should be stored in a dark place, and the vials should only be non-transparent glass. Keep them away from heat sources in order to preserve their concentration and efficiency.

Essential oils can be integrated into cosmetic formulas and body lotions as well as shower gels.

EXAMPLE OF A PREPARATION FOR A BODY MASSAGE OIL:

If you want to make your massage oil at home and for yourself, here are the basic ingredients:

- One 50 ml non-transparent glass bottle
- 5 drops of essential oils of your choice.
- 50 ml of massage oil of your choice.
- You can use two kinds of essential oils.

ESSENTIAL OILS, THEIR COMPOSITION AND USES:

Essential oils are extracted from unique and natural essences of certain aromatic plants, trees, fruits, flowers, herbs and spices.

There are more than 150 pure and concentrated essential oils, whose effects are optimal and beneficial thanks to their aroma concentration.

Each of the essential oils may contain more than 100 active chemicals.

Essential oils can be used individually or combined.

It is vital to choose the right essential oils to optimize their synergies, results and benefits in order to avoid allergic skin reactions. Generally, you can use 3 or 4 essential oils in the same formula, provided you choose them according to their synergy and harmony.

ESSENTIAL OILS AND PRECAUTIONS OF USE:

Essential oils can be incorporated into cosmetic formulas and body lotions.

They can also be used in liquid soaps.

- Avoid using essential oils around the eyes.
- Do not use essential oils if you are pregnant.
- Avoid essential oils on irritated skin.
- Essential oils are prohibited on people at medical risk.

- Keep essential oils out of reach of children.
- Not for babies.
- Essential oils should be stored in a dark place.
- The bottles must imperatively be non-transparent.
- Keep essential oils away from heat in order to maintain their effectiveness.
- It is imperative to follow their instructions for use and dosage in order to preserve the safety and optimization of the essential oils in your formula.
- The properties of essential oils are diverse: they are invigorating, anti-stress, soothing, stimulating and relaxing.

LIST OF COSMETIC ESSENTIAL OILS:

- Sage essential oil
- lime essential oil
- mint and peppermint essential oil
- lavender essential oil
- lang yang essential oil
- yellow sandalwood essential oil
- helichrysum essential oil
- eucalyptus essential oil
- cypress essential oil
- sweet orange essential oil
- palmarosa essential oil
- Ravensara essential oil
- cedarwood essential oil
- geranium essential oil
- carrot essential oil
- grapefruit essential oil
- verbena essential oil
- sweet almond essential oil
- balsam essential oil
- coriander essential oil
- tea tree essential oil
- lemon essential oil
- marjoram essential oil
- patchouli essential oil
- palmarosa essential oil
- chamomile essential oil
- ginger essential oil
- sage essential oil
- geranium essential oil
- bergamot essential oil
- Niaouli essential oil
- cinnamon essential oil
- vetiver essential oil
- cedar essential oil
- organic aloe Vera essential oil.

CHAPTER 6

Floral Waters Or Hydrosols

Hydrosol floral water is concentrated in active ingredients and belongs to the realm of aromatherapy.

Hydrosol floral water is a fragile tonic.

It should be stored in an opaque bottle and kept in the refrigerator.

Its conservation cannot exceed 2 months.

Hydrosol floral waters are generally used as a tonic, they can also be incorporated in face and body beauty creams and milks.

The production of hydrosol floral water is easy and inexpensive.

Use fresh or dry flowers and plants.

The aroma will be more accentuated with fresh flowers and plants.

Hydrosol floral water comes from the distillation of water transformed into vapor from plants or flowers.

Their qualities and properties are similar to essential oils, but their concentration is low, which allows a wider aromatic for all ages and skin types (not for children and babies).

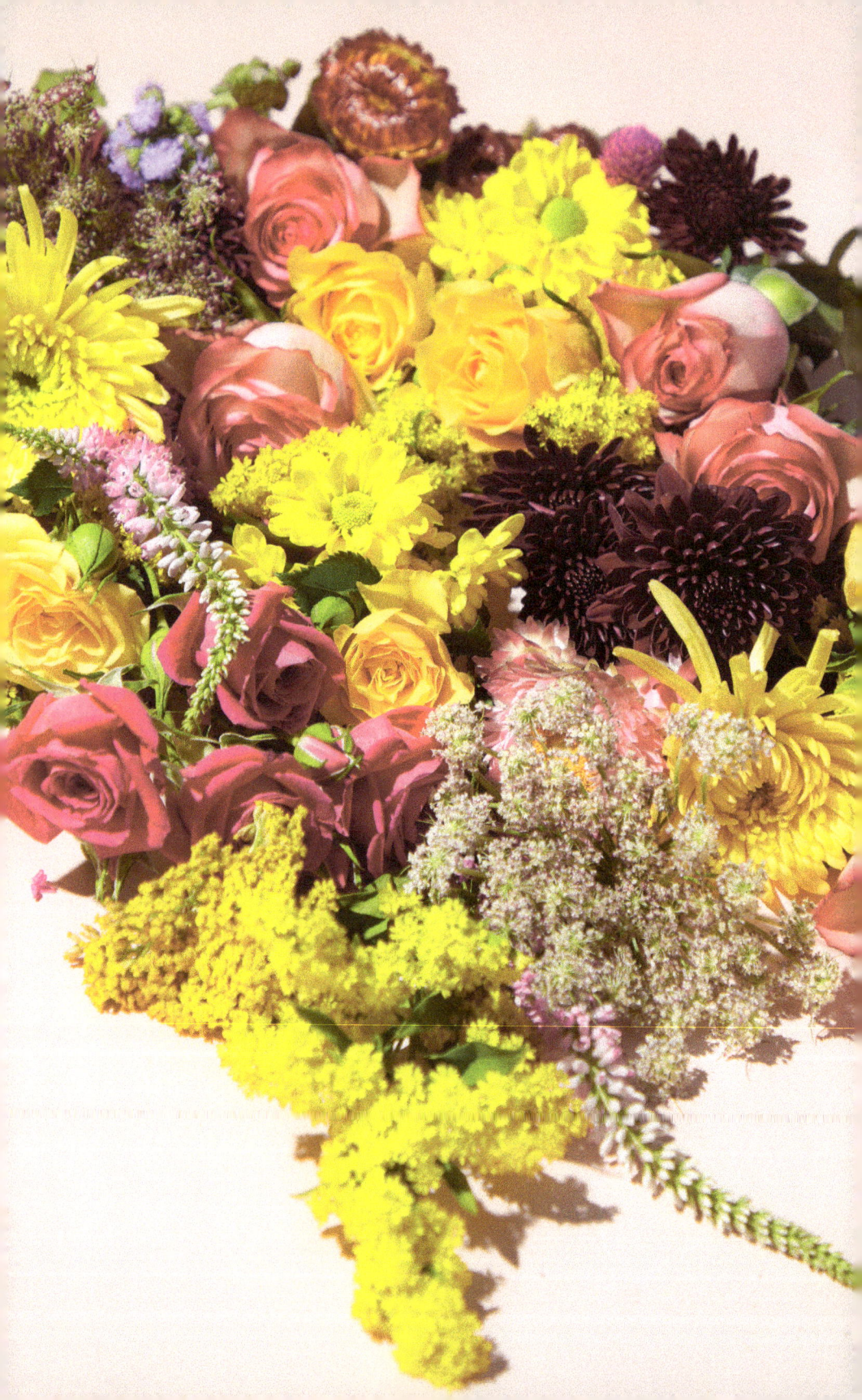

LIST OF PLANTS AND FLOWERS TO USE IN FLORAL WATER HYDROSOLS:

BLUEBERRY WATER:

It is a hydrosol floral water with calming and decongesting effects.

ORANGE BLOSSOM:

It is an invigorating hydrosol floral water; it may relieve tired eyes and may reduce bags under the eyes.

ROSE WATER:

It is a hydrosol floral water very often used in tonics.

It softens, hydrates, decongests and evens out the skin.

PEPPERMINT:

It is a hydrosol floral water with invigorating effects. It helps the skin recover its radiance and improves skin circulation.

THE ALOE VERA PLANT:

A floral water rich in vitamins. It is calming and rich in trace elements.

CLAYS: LIST OF CLAYS USED IN COSMETICS:

There exist different clays used to make different kinds of face masks.

GREEN CLAY:

This is the most famous clay used in face masks. It is suitable for oily, combination skin. It has calming properties.

WHITE CLAY: (ALSO CALLED KAOLIN):

It is recommended for sensitive and irritated skin; it softens the skin and may regulate sebum.

RED CLAY:

It restores the skin's luminous appearance and is recommended for skins with a dull complexion.

CHAPTER 7

How To Make Your Beauty Products At Home

Making your beauty products at home means creating your own workshop with the scents, textures and benefits you look for, using the natural scents of essential oils or organic flavors.

You can also plan a budget in choosing the ingredients that suit your skin type.

It also allows you to get in a good habit of knowing and choosing the ingredients that seem best suited to your skin type, while respecting the dosage and the qualitative ingredients that correspond to your skin type.

Making your beauty products at home represents a 20% investment compared to the price of cosmetics bought in stores.

RULES TO FOLLOW IN MAKING YOUR OWN PRODUCTS:

Your homemade cosmetic products require certain rules to be respected.

- Hygiene, to avoid bacteria.
- Safety instructions and disinfection of tools / equipment.
- Label the products with a label indicating the date of their production, the date of their expiry.
- Disposable gloves are a must.
- It is recommended to use a few drops of natural preservatives such as: wheat germ oil or vitamin E.
- When you create your lip balm you must keep it cool and away from air, light and heat.
- For hydrosols: in general, they can be stored in the fridge and remain compatible for 3-6 months (provided that you add vitamin E to your hydrosols, which is the best natural preservative.

TEST YOUR FINISHED PRODUCTS ON YOUR SKIN:

Your formulas contain essential oils and vegetable oils which can cause allergic reactions.

The test is carried out: 1 drop of cream in the hollow of the inside of the elbow.

Keep the cream for 12 hours before rinsing. If your skin reddens, then reduce your dosage of essential oils.

Respect the dosage of the ingredients of each of the formulas. before starting the realization of your cosmetic products, it is vital to bring together all the instruments / equipment, the work plan, sterilize them with 90% alcohol.

LIST OF MATERIALS TO HAVE BEFORE MAKING YOUR PRODUCTS:

- 1 small whisk / spatula / mini mixer
- 1 medium size bowl.
- 1 pipette.
- 1 measuring spoon.
- 1 small funnel.

- ⌒ 1 small saucepan.
- ⌒ 1 pair of scissors.

- ⌒ 1 knife.

PREPARE THE INGREDIENTS IN ADVANCE:

- ⌒ Essential oils.
- ⌒ Vegetable oils.
- ⌒ Hydrosols or floral waters.

- ⌒ The list of fruits and vegetables needed for each of your formulas.

HOW TO MAKE YOUR BEAUTY PRODUCTS AT HOME WITH ORGANIC INGREDIENTS:

REMEMBER:

A beauty cream recipe with organic ingredients has a very limited shelf life.

It is necessary systematically to stick and note on the label: the date of production and of the potting of the product (creams, lotions, etc.).

It is imperative to adapt the formula of your cream / lotion to the type of skin

(oily, dry, combination…).

In general, beauty products made from organic ingredients may last for one month (provided the finished product is saved in the fridge).

In general, all organic vegetable oils can be used in your formulas. At the end of each of the formulas you can add a few drops of vitamin E oil, which maintains the stability and longevity of the formula.

PRECAUTIONS TO BE TAKEN WHEN USING ORGANIC ESSENTIAL OILS:

It is important to follow the instructions for use and the recommended dosage for a safe obtaining of your formula.

LIST OF ESSENTIAL OILS:

- The properties of essential oils are various, invigorating, anti-stress,
- Soothing, stimulating, relaxing.

LIST OF ESSENTIAL OILS USED IN COSMETICS:

- SAGE essential oil.
- Lemon / lime essential oil.
- Mint essential oil, peppermint.
- Lavender essential oil.
- Yang essential oil.
- Yellow sandalwood essential oil.
- Helichrysum essential oil– Eucalyptus essential oil.
- Cypress essential oil.
- Sweet orange essential oil.
- Palmarosa essential oil.
- Ravensara essential oil– Cedarwood essential oil.
- Sweet orange essential oil.
- Geranium essential oil.
- Carrot essential oil.
- Grapefruit essential oil.
- Verbena essential oil.
- Sweet almond essential oil.
- Balsam fir essential oil. coriander essential oil.

6 NATURAL INGREDIENTS WHICH MAY HELP WITH A COLD SORE/HERPES:

It is painful.

It might be possible to alleviate its symptoms and relieve the pain with some natural ingredients.

THE LIST OF NATURAL INGREDIENTS THAT MAY HELP WITH HERPES:

- 1 Tea Tree essential oil.
- 2 Niaouli essential oil.
- 3 Green clay paste.
- 4 Organic honey.
- 5 Ice cubes.
- Organic cider vinegar.

THE FORMULAS OF HOMEMADE CREAMS:

A BASIC NOTION:

In order to obtain a cream, it is necessary to combine an aqueous phase and a greasy phase.

The first phase, aqueous, uses a few large spoons of mineral or—preferably—floral water.

The second phase generally includes vegetable oils or essential oils, beeswax or vegetable butters.

In the 2 complementary phases, one hydrates and the second phase nurish.

It is necessary to emulsify them to obtain a homogeneous and smooth cream.

LIST OF COSMETIC ACTIVE INGREDIENTS THAT YOU CAN USE IN THE PREPARATION OF YOUR HOMEMADE FORMULAS:

- 1 Organic beech bud extract (may help preserves youthfulness).
- 2 The liquid organic Silicon.
- 3 Liquid rice protein (for a moisturizing effect).
- 4 Provitamin B5 (panthenol, and soothing properties).
- 5 Liquid marshmallow flower extract (for moisturizing effect).
- 6 Organic orchid extract (rich in antioxidants and for mature skin).
- 7 Powdered ginseng extract (firming effect).
- 8 Organic plant extract (for body care).
- 9 Stabilized vitamin C powder (stimulates collagen, radiance of the complexion).
- 10 Organic aloe vera powder.
- 11 Coconut milk powder (rich in fatty acids,

vitamins, excellent for the skin and the body for tired skin).

- 12 Sweet almond milk powder.

- 13 Keratin cosmetic active ingredient based on brown algae extracts.

- 14 Active elastin booster (stimulates elastin synthesis, restores the tonus of the skin).

- 15 Active cosmetic DHA natural (can be added in creams in order to give a self-tanning effect to the skin).

- 16 Plant collagen and yeast extract together (they smooth the skin).

- 17 Activated vegetable carbon (with detoxifying properties).

- 18 Allantoin active ingredient (softening, soothing active ingredient).

- 19 Plant salicylic acid extract (is a cosmetic active ingredient for skins oily and acne-prone).

- 20 glycolic acid

- 21 Papaya powder (rich in enzymes, niche in vitamins, moisturizing.

- 22 Pumpkin vegetable powder, rich in enzymes, vitamins A, B, C, E.

- Regulates cutaneous sebum, rich in zinc and potassium.

- 23 Powder of blueberry and raspberry, rich in vitamins F, A, C, B6, and zinc. rich in antioxidants, powerful for the skin, rich in oxygen supply for the skin.

- Organic grenadine juice, powerful antioxidant, contains Retinol, rich in antioxidants, in collagen, may fill out wrinkles.

CHAPTER 8

Recipes

Lotions, Tonics, and Make-up Removers

1. TONIC FOR NORMAL, COMBINATION SKIN

MATERIAL:

- 1 PET 100 ml spray bottle

INGREDIENTS:

- 80 ml of mineral water / floral water of your choice.
- 5 ml of vegetable glycerin.
- 2 large spoons of liquid bamboo plant extract.
- 2 small spoons of organic aloe Vera gel.
- 5 mg of powder of Ayurvedic plants.
- 1/2 teaspoon of liquid bamboo extract.
- 20 drops of Cosgard preservative / 10 drops of vitamin E.

INSTRUCTIONS FOR USE:

- Pour all the ingredients into the bottle.
- Close the bottle tightly, shake the bottle for 3 minutes.
- Use this tonic every night by spraying it on your face and neck. let the tonic dry on the skin, and then use an evening cream.

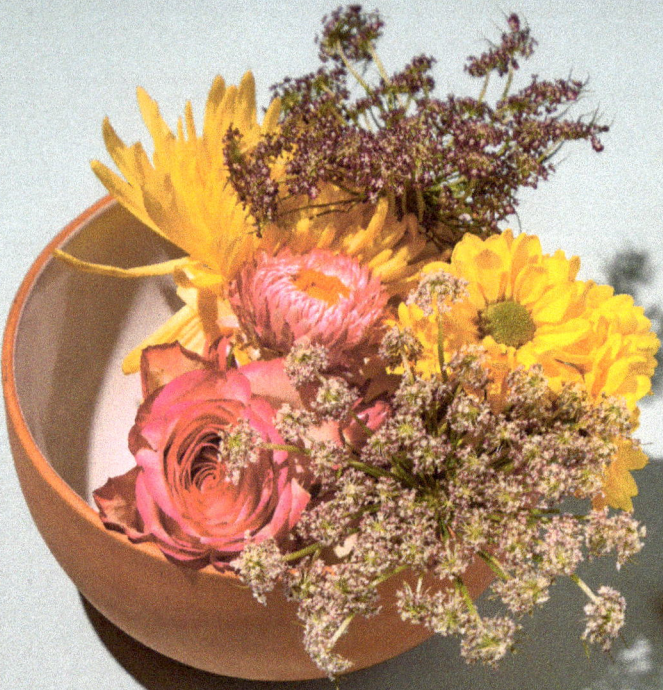

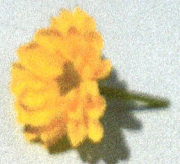

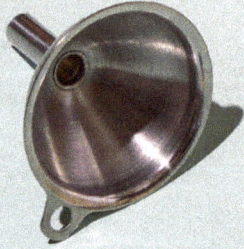

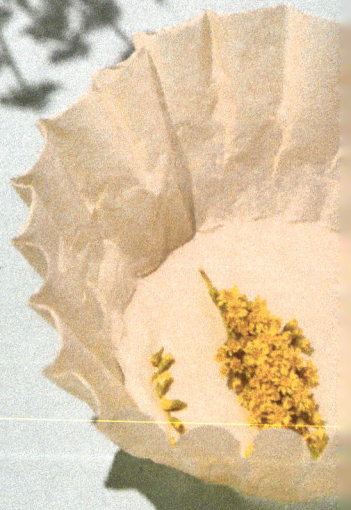

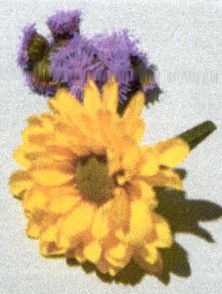

2. BEAUTY RECIPES TONING LOTIONS: HOW TO MAKE YOUR FLORAL WATER-HYDROLATE AT HOME

HERE ARE 2 PREPARATION MODES:

NO. 1, EASY AND QUICK TO MAKE:

MATERIAL:

- 1 400 ml saucepan.
- 1 medium bowl.
- 1 paper coffee filter.
- 1 250 ml glass spray bottle or in PET.
- 1 small funnel.

INGREDIENTS:

- 250 g of fresh or dried flowers or plants.
- 4 capsules of vitamin E.
- 400 ml of water.

INSTRUCTIONS FOR USE:

- Pour the water into the pan, heat the water. Turn off the heat before the water boils.
- Place the plants or flowers in the bowl.
- Carefully pour hot water over the plants in the bowl.
- Cover the bowl. Let the plants macerate in the bowl for 1 hour.
- Filter the water in the bowl. Let cool.
- Place the coffee filter in, and then place the funnel at the top of the bottle.
- Pour the floral water into the funnel filter.
- Add vitamin E to the bottle. Shake the bottle well and keep the bottle in the fridge.

- NOTE: all floral waters
- Homemade hydrosols can be kept for 2 months

provided they are kept in the refrigerator

NO 2: MATERIAL:

- 1 pot steamer, (composed of 3 parts).
- 1 funnel.
- 1 250 ml glass spray bottle or PET.

INGREDIENTS:

- 400 ml of water.
- 250 g of fresh or dried plants.
- 4 drops of vitamin E.

INSTRUCTIONS FOR USE:

- Pour the water into the pot steamer, (in the bottom part)
- .Place the 2nd part of the pot steamer, (the strainer.)
- Place the plants or flowers on top of the strainer.
- . Place the small tray in the middle of the plants.
- Cover the steamer (place the lid upside down).
- Place a layer of ice cubes on the upside down lid.
- Adjust the thermostat for 30 minutes.
- Let the pot steamer cool. Remove the cover.
- Collect the small tray with the floral water-hydrosol.
- Using the funnel, pour the floral water into the bottle.
- Add 4 drops of vitamin E to the bottle. Store the bottle in the refrigerator.
- Shake the bottle well before each use of this tonic.

3. TONING RECIPE FOR ALL SKIN TYPES

INGREDIENTS:

- 1 small 50 ml glass bottle.
- 1/4 glass of organic aloe vera water.
- 1 small spoonful of rose water.
- 10 large spoons of fresh cucumber juice. juice of 1/2 of a freshly squeezed lemon.

INSTRUCTIONS FOR USE:

- Peel the cucumber, grate it and strain it out to collect it water.
- Pour all the ingredients into the bottle. Keep the bottle in the fridge.
- Every morning uses this tonic to cleanse and refresh your skin.

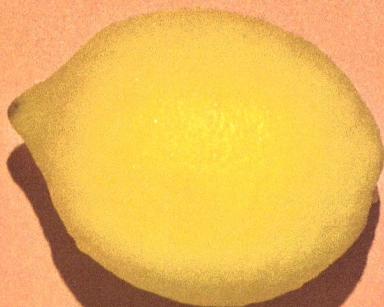

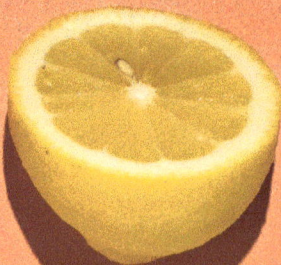

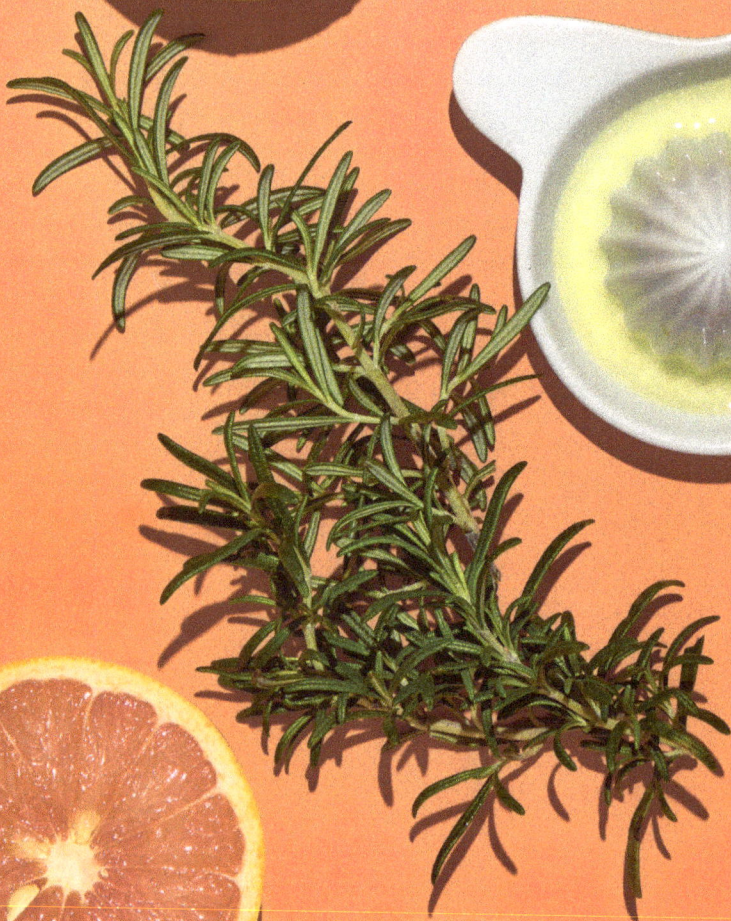

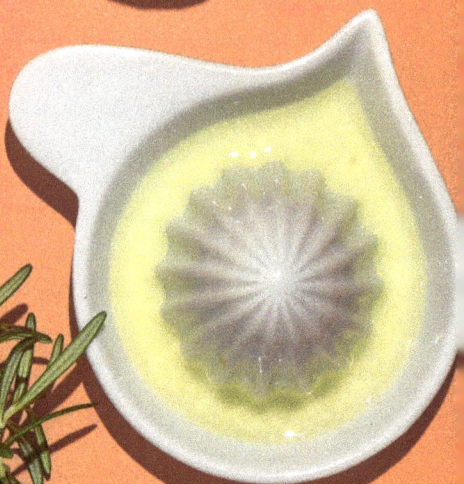

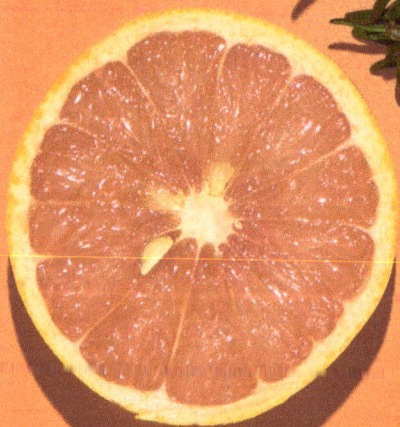

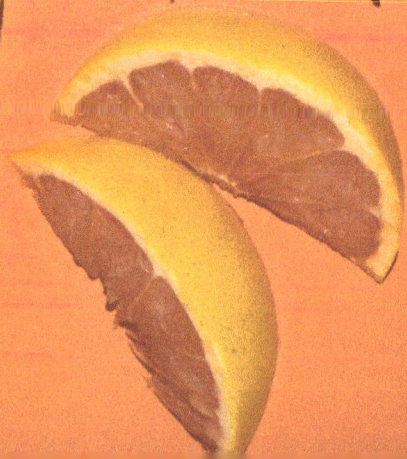

4. FACE TONIC WITH PLANTS FOR OILY SKIN

INGREDIENTS:

- 1 250g glass bottle/ PET.
- 1 medium saucepan.
- 25 g of rosemary leaves, fresh and dried.
- 1/4 liters of water.
- 1 large spoon of freshly squeezed lemon juice.
- 5 drops of grapefruit essential oil.
- 2 drops of vitamin E.

INSTRUCTIONS FOR USE:

- Pour the water into the saucepan, add the rosemary leaves.
- Bring to a boil for 5 minutes.
- Remove the pan from the heat. Let cool.
- Filter the water, and then pour the water into the bottle.
- Add the remaining ingredients to the bottle.
- Close the bottle tightly. Shake the bottle well for 1 minute.
- Using a compress, use this tonic to cleanse the face.
- Use the tonic 2 times a day.
- This tonic should be kept in the refrigerator for 2 weeks.

5.   PLANT TONIC FOR DRY / IRRITATED SKIN

INGREDIENTS:

- 1 small saucepan.
- 1 strainer.
- 1 250ml bottle.
- 200 ml of water.
- 30 g of fresh and dried lime leaves.
- 1 teaspoon of evening primrose / almond oil.
- 5 drops of blueberry essential oil.
- 5 drops of chamomile essential oil

DIRECTIONS:

- In the saucepan, pour the linden leaves with 250 ml of water.
- Let boil for 10 minutes.
- Filter the water. Let cool.
- Pour the water into the bottle. Add the oils.
- Using a compress soaked in this tonic, cleanse your face and neck 2 times a day.
- This tonic should be kept in the refrigerator for a period of use limited to 15 days.

6. PURIFYING AYURVEDIC FACE TONIC

MATERIAL:

- 1 mini whisk / spatula.
- 1 small funnel.
- 1 paper coffee filter.
- 1 glass spray bottle of 50 ml / PET.
- 1 medium bowl.

INGREDIENTS:

- 20 ml of mineral water or rose water.
- 25 ml of linden / geranium hydrosol.
- 1/2 teaspoon of organic Aloe vera powder.
- 1/2 spoon of organic Ayurvedic Amla plant powder.
- 1/4 teaspoon of baking soda powder.
- 7 drops of lemon essential oil.

INSTRUCTIONS FOR USE:

- Pour the baking soda powder, the aloe vera, the Ayurvedic Amla herbal powder into the bowl.
- Pour the geranium hydrosol or linden water / blueberry water into the bowl.
- Mix all the ingredients in the bowl using the whisk.
- Let this preparation sit for 12 hours.
- With the coffee filter, filter the tonic.
- Using the funnel, pour the tonic into the bottle.
- Add the lemon / mandarin essential oils to the bottle.
- Close the bottle and shake it before each use.
- Use tonic spray in the evening after your makeup removal.

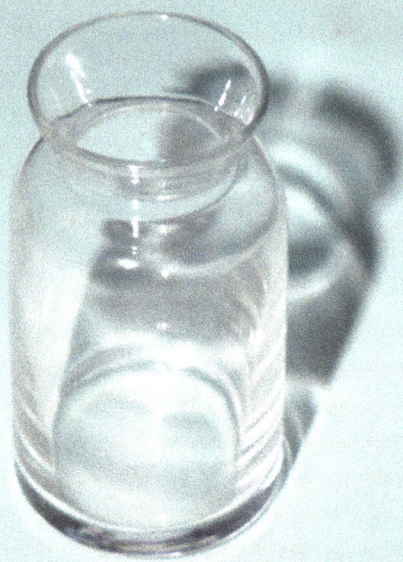

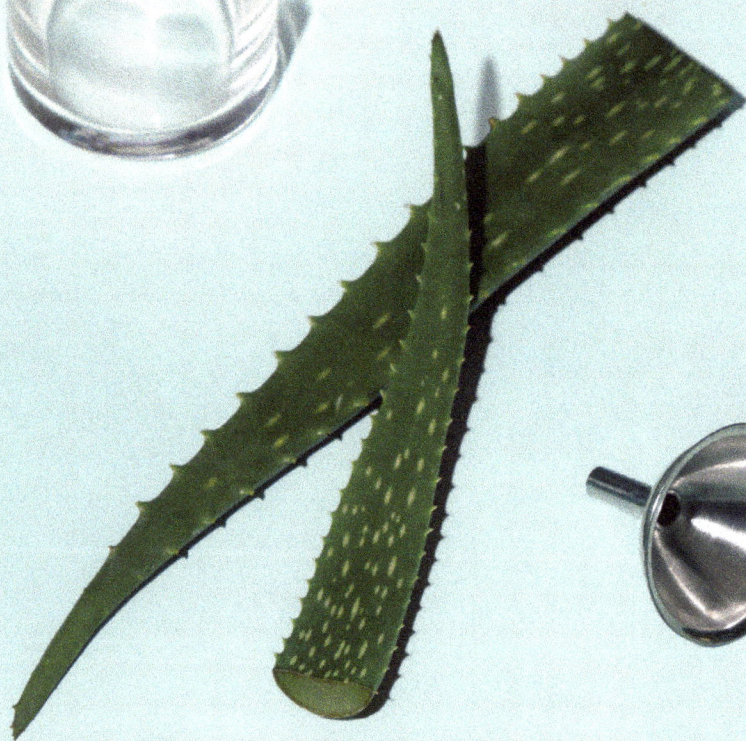

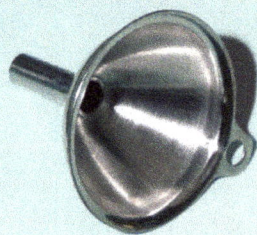

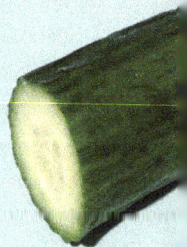

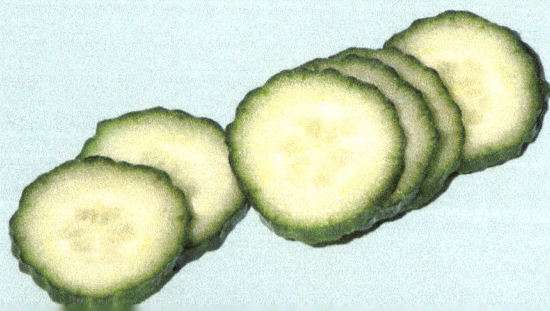

7.   CUCUMBER TONIC FOR ALL SKIN

MATERIAL:

- 1 50ml glass spray bottle.
- 1 large sterile compress. small funnel.

INGREDIENTS:

- 1/4 glass of organic aloe Vera water.
- 1 teaspoon of rose water.
- 10 large spoons of filtered fresh cucumber juice.
- Juice of 1/2 of a freshly squeezed lemon.

INSTRUCTIONS FOR USE:

- Peel 1 large cucumber and grate it.
- Open the large compress, place the grated cucumber into it.
- Close the compress and wring it out to collect the juice from the cucumber.
- Pour all the ingredients into the bottle.
- Before using this tonic, thoroughly remove make-up from your skin, then spray your skin with this tonic. Store the vial in the refrigerator.

8. BLUEBERRY AND CHAMOMILE MAKEUP REMOVER

MATERIAL:

- 1 small saucepan.
- 1 small strainer.
- 1 small funnel.
- 1 glass bottle of 100 ml.

INGREDIENTS:

- 100 g of dried chamomile flowers.
- 30 ml of mineral water.
- 50 ml of blueberry water or blueberry macerate.
- 20 ml of organic jojoba vegetable oil / rosemary macerate oil.

DIRECTIONS:

- Pour the dried chamomile flowers into the saucepan.
- Pour 30 ml of mineral water in the pan, cover the pan. boil for 5-7 minutes.
- Remove the pan from the heat. Let cool.
- With the colander, filter the chamomile water.
- Using the funnel, pour into the flask.
- Add the rest of the ingredients to the bottle.
- Close the bottle, shake it well before use.
- It is recommended to use compresses to remove makeup.

9. PLANT TONIC FOR ALL SKINS

MATERIAL:

- 1 small saucepan.
- 1 bottle of 50 ml.
- 1 colander.
- 1 small funnel.

INGREDIENTS:

- 2 large cups of mineral water.
- 3 large spoons of fresh or dried chamomile leaves.
- 3 large spoons of fresh or dry mint leaves.
- 2 large spoons of fresh or dried verbena leaves.
- 2 drops of Ravensara / verbena essential oil.

DIRECTIONS:

- Pour the plants and water into the pot.
- Put the pan on the heat, let it boil for 5 minutes.
- Remove the pan from the heat. Let cool.
- Using the colander, filter the tonic.
- Using the funnel, pour the water into the bottle.
- Close the bottle tightly, shake it well before each use.
- Use this tonic after each make-up removal.

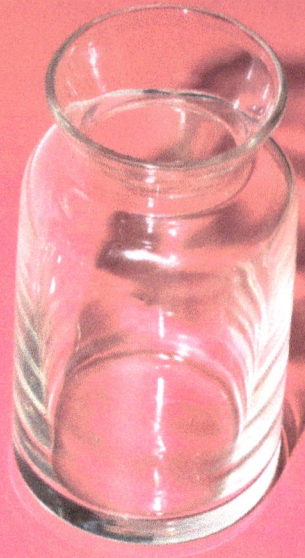

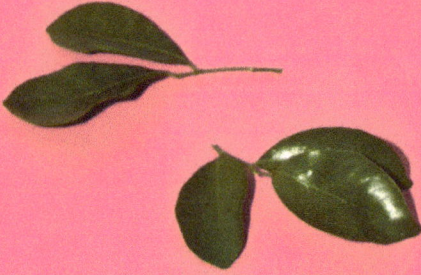

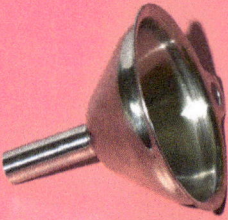

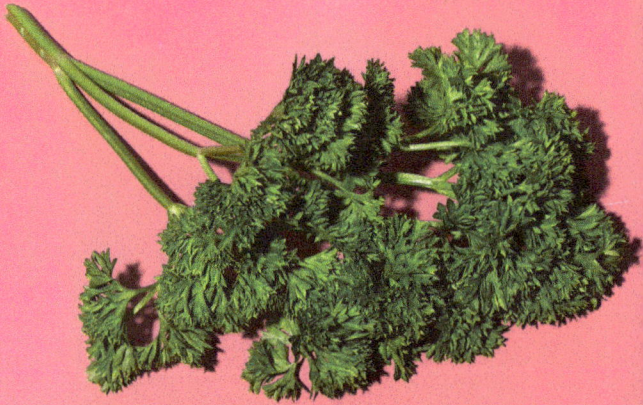

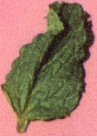

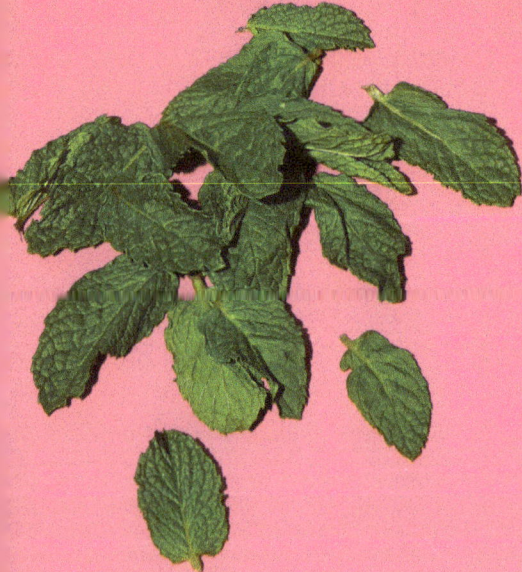

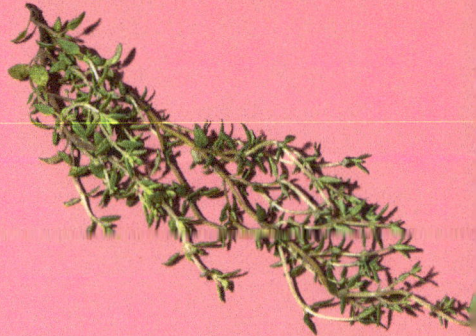

10. SCRAPING TONIC FOR DILATED PORES

MATERIAL:

- 1 small saucepan.
- 1 glass bottle of 100 ml.
- 1 colander.
- 1 small funnel.

INGREDIENTS:

- 2 large cups of mineral water.
- 10 dried lemon balm leaves.
- 2 sprigs of fresh thyme.
- 20 leaves of fresh mint.
- 10 branches of fresh parsley leaves.

INSTRUCTIONS FOR USE:

- Place all the ingredients in the small saucepan.
- Carefully pour 2 large cups of boiling water into the saucepan.
- Leave to stand overnight.
- In the morning, using the colander, filter the water.
- Using the funnel, pour the lotion into the bottle.
- Shake the bottle well before each use.
- Keep this tonic in the refrigerator.

11. MINT AND FRESH BASIL TONIC

MATERIAL:

- 1 spray bottle of 100 ml in glass or PET.
- 1 small saucepan.
- 1 colander.
- 1 scissors.
- 1 spatula.

INGREDIENTS:

- 30 leaves of fresh basil.
- 45 leaves of fresh mint.
- 2 medium cups of mineral water.
- 2 drops of vitamin E.

INSTRUCTIONS FOR USE:

- Using scissors, cut the basil and mint leaves into small pieces.
- Pour the 2 medium cups of water into the saucepan.
- Place the pan on the heat, let it boil for 2 minutes.
- Remove the pan from the heat. Let cool.
- Using the colander, filter the tonic infusion.
- Using the funnel, pour the tonic infusion into the bottle.
- Add vitamin E. to the bottle.
- Use this tonic in the evening after removing make-up from the skin.
- Store this tonic in the refrigerator.

12. TONIC FOR DRY SKIN

MATERIAL:

- 1 bottle of 50 ml of spray in glass or PET.
- 1 sterile empty pipette of 50 ml.

INGREDIENTS:

- 15 ml of lavender or chamomile hydrosol.
- 10 ml of cornflower water or rose water.
- 15 drops of carrot essential oil.
- 5 drops of sandalwood / orange essential oil.
- 2 drops of organic glycerin.
- 2 drops of vitamin E.

INSTRUCTIONS FOR USE:

- Using the pipette, pour all the ingredients into the bottle.
- Close the bottle, shake it well before each use. store the vial in a cool place (not in the refrigerator).

13. PLANT TONIC FOR OILY AND COMBINATION SKIN

MATERIAL:

- 1 small saucepan.
- 1 small colander.
- 1 bottle of 250ml in spray glass.

INGREDIENTS:

- 25 g of fresh or dried rosemary leaves.
- 1/4 liter of water.
- 1 large spoon of fresh squeezed lemon juice.
- 5 drops of grapefruit essential oil.
- 2 drops of vitamin E.

INSTRUCTIONS FOR USE:

- Pour the water into the saucepan. Add the rosemary leaves.
- Bring to the boil for 10 minutes.
- Remove the pan from the fire. Let cool.
- Filter the infusion and pour it into the bottle.
- Add the rest of the ingredients to the bottle. Shake the bottle well.
- Soak a compress in this tonic to refresh your face.
- You can use this tonic up to 2 times / day.
- Store this tonic in the refrigerator (maximum 2 months).

14. PLANT TONIC FOR DRY AND IRRITATED SKIN

MATERIAL:

- 1 small saucepan.
- 1 small colander.
- 1 glass bottle of 250 ml.

INGREDIENTS:

- 200 ml of water.
- 30g of fresh or dried lime leaves.
- 1 teaspoon of evening primrose / almond vegetable oil.
- 10 drops of cornflower essential oil.
- 10 drops of chamomile essential oil.

INSTRUCTIONS FOR USE:

- Pour the lime leaves and 250 ml of water into the saucepan.
- Place the pan on the heat. Let boil for 10 minutes.
- Remove the pan from the heat. Let cool.
- Using the colander, filter the infusion.
- Using the funnel, pour the infusion into the bottle.
- Add the essential oils to the bottle. Shake the bottle well before each use.
- Soak a compress with this tonic after each make-up removal.
- You can store your tonic in the refrigerator for a period of 2 weeks.

15. MAKE-UP REMOVER COMBINATION FOR SKIN WITH LIQUID EXTRACT OF MARSHMALLOW FLOWERS

MATERIAL:

- 1 PET spray bottle of 100 ml.
- 1 stainless steel spatula.
- 1 small funnel.

INGREDIENTS:

- 20 ml of tea tree hydrosol / chamomile water.
- 40 ml of mineral water.
- 25 ml of liquid extract of marshmallow flowers / liquid extract of flowers organic orchid.
- 2 small spoons of cosmetic active extract of allantoin.
- 1/2 teaspoon of baking soda powder.

INSTRUCTIONS FOR USE:

- Pour all the ingredients into the bottle.
- Close the bottle tightly, shake it well for 2 minutes.
- Use this makeup remover morning and night.

16. ROSEMARY TONIC FOR ALL SKIN

MATERIAL:
- 1 250 ml PET spray bottle.

INGREDIENTS:
- 220 ml of floral water / plant hydrosol.
- 10 drops of glycerin
- 20 ml of organic vegetable collagen gel / liquid ginger extract.
- 5 drops of grapefruit essential oil.
- 10 drops of chamomile essential oil.

INSTRUCTIONS FOR USE:
- Pour all the ingredients into the bottle.
- Close the bottle tightly, then shake it for 3 minutes.
- Place the bottle in a place at room temperature (bathroom).
- Leave the bottle to stand for 5 days.
- Before each use, shake the bottle well.
- Spray your face and neck with this lotion. Leave to dry.
- Use your day / evening cream.

17. BASIL AND MINT LEAVES TONIC FOR ALL SKIN

MATERIAL:

- 1 small saucepan.
- 1 small colander.
- 1 100ml spray bottle.

INGREDIENTS:

- 15 leaves of fresh or dried basil.
- 10 fresh or dried mint leaves.
- 10 fresh or dried verbena leaves.
- 2 cups of boiling water.
- 2 drops of zinc
- 4 drops of liquid extract of marshmallow / cornflower flowers.
- 2 drops of organic glycerin oil.
- 10 ml of organic avocado vegetable oil.
- 3 drops of rose essential oil.

INSTRUCTIONS FOR USE:

- Cut the leaves of the plants. Pour them into the small saucepan.
- Add the 2 cups of boiling water to the saucepan.
- Place the pan on the heat. Let boil for 2 minutes.
- Carefully remove the pan from the heat. Let cool.
- Using the colander, filter the water from the plants.
- Let it cool, then pour this plant water into the spray bottle.
- Add the rest of the ingredients to the bottle.
- Close the bottle tightly, shake it for 1 minute.
- Use this spray lotion on the skin after makeup removal.
- Let the skin dry. Then use a cream containing vitamin C '

18. BLUEBERRY AND CHAMOMILE MAKE-UP REMOVER

INGREDIENTS:

- 1 bottle of 100 ml in glass / PET.
- 100 g of dried chamomile flowers.
- 60 ml of mineral water.
- 40 ml of blueberry water / blueberry macerate.
- 25 ml of organic avocado / sesame vegetable oil.

DIRECTIONS:

- Pour the dried chamomile flowers into a small saucepan.
- Pour 60 ml of mineral water over the chamomile flowers. Cover the pan. Let it boil for 5-7 minutes.
- Remove the pan from the heat. Let cool. Using a colander, filter and collect the water from the chamomile.
- Pour the chamomile water into the bottle. Add the rest the bottle of the ingredients too. Close the bottle. Shake the bottle well before each use. Use only compresses to remove makeup.

19. REFRESHING FACE GEL FOR ALL SKINS

MATERIAL:

- 1 glass bottle of 50 ml.

INGREDIENTS:

- 10 ml of linseed oil / apricot kernels.
- 35 ml of organic aloe Vera gel.
- 10 drops of essential oil of seeds grapefruit.
- 5 drops of linden essential oil.

INSTRUCTIONS FOR USE:

- Pour all the ingredients into the bottle.
- Close the bottle tightly, and shake it for 1 minute.
- Before each use, shake the bottle well.
- Use this gel as a day care 4 times / week.

Day Creams
and Night Creams

20. ANTI AGING CREAM

MATERIAL:

- 1 medium bowl.
- 1 spatula
- 1 glass jar of 100ml.

INGREDIENTS:

- 30 ml of organic avocado vegetable oil.
- 60 ml of blueberry water / plant hydrosol.
- 2 drops of hyaluronic acid.
- 2 drops of vitamin E.
- 10 drops of verbena essential oil.
- 10 drops of beech bud extract / 5 drop of organic silicon.
- 5 drops of liquid rice protein.
- 1/4 teaspoon of organic Aloe vera powder.

DIRECTIONS:

- Mix in the bowl: avocado oil + plant hydrosol / blueberry water. place the bowl in a bain-marie, while continuing to mix with the spatula until a uniform whitish cream is obtained.
- Add the hyaluronic acid.
- Remove the bowl from the bain-marie.
- Place the bowl in a small basin of cold water.
- Add the remaining ingredients to the bowl, continue mixing for 1 minute.
- Pour the cream into the pot. Close the jar and store the jar of cream in the refrigerator.
- Use this night cream 3 times / week alternating with a conventional cream.

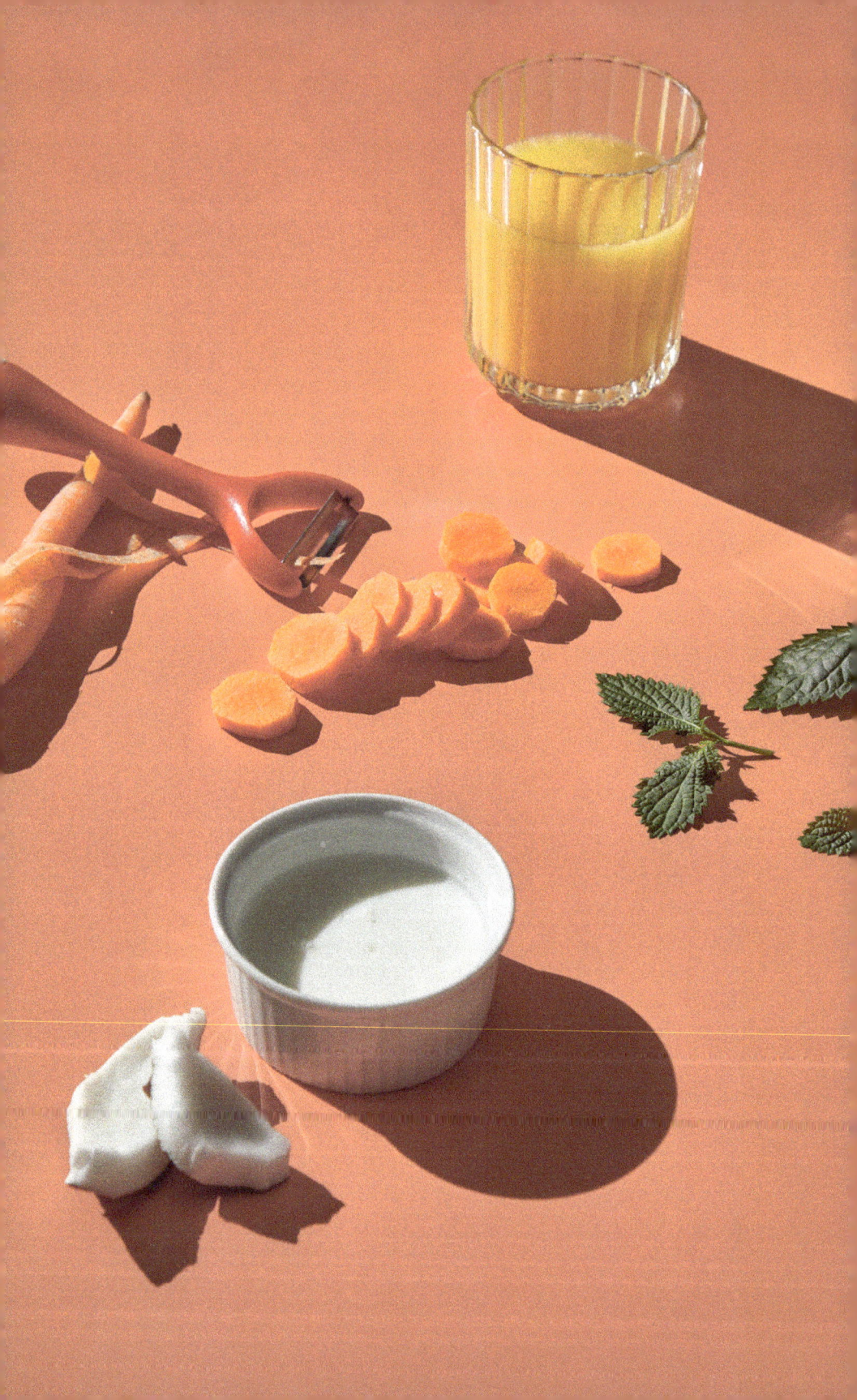

21. COCONUT MILK AND VERBENA DAY CREAM

MATERIAL:

- 1 medium bowl.
- 1 glass jar of 100 ml.
- 1 wooden spatula.

INGREDIENTS:

- 10 ml of carrot vegetable oil.
- 60 ml of plant hydrosol / orange blossom water.
- 10 ml of organic coconut milk.
- 1/4 of a teaspoon of gelatin active powder.
- 1 teaspoon of organic glycerin.
- 10 drops of verbena essential oil.

INSTRUCTIONS FOR USE:

- Pour all the ingredients into the bowl.
- Place the bowl in the Marie bath.
- Using the spatula, mix all the ingredients for 3 minutes in the bowl until a smooth, fluid cream is obtained.
- Remove the bowl from the bain-marie and pour the cream into the pot.
- Close the jar and store the cream in the refrigerator.
- Use this cream 3 times / week alternating with a conventional cream.

22. POST SUN, CREAM WHICH MAY HELP CALM SUNBURNS

MATERIAL:

- 1 small spatula.
- 1 empty glass cream jar of 100ml.

INGREDIENTS:

- 1/2 fresh yogurt.
- 7 drops of chamomile essential oil.
- 7 drops of lavender essential oil.
- 1 teaspoon of organic aloe Vera gel.
- 3 drops of vitamin E oil.– 10 drops of Tamanu oil.

INSTRUCTIONS FOR USE:

- Pour all the ingredients into the pot.
- Using the small spatula, mix all the ingredients well until obtained a smooth, fluid cream is.
- Using the small spatula, apply the cream to the sunburned areas of the skin.
- Let me act for 7-8 minutes.
- Rinse with cool water.

23. GOOD GLOW DAY CREAM FOR ALL SKIN TYPES

MATERIAL:

- 2 medium bowls.
- 1 small whisk.
- 1 empty 15 ml syringe.
- 1 bottle / jar of 100 ml.

INGREDIENTS:

PHASE 1:

- 15 ml of oily macerate of carrots / avocado oil.
- 15 ml of vegetable oil of hazelnuts / apricots.
- 7 small spoons of neutral gel / organic aloe vera.

PHASE 2:

- 80 ml of witch hazel / blueberry hydrosol.

PHASE 3:

- 15 drops of verbena / chamomile essential oil.
- 1 teaspoon of organic glycerin oil.
- 20 drops of cosgard preservative or 5 drops of vitamin E.

INSTRUCTIONS FOR USE:

POUR INTO BOWL No1:

- macerated water of carrots / vegetable oil of apricots / hazelnut oil.

- Add to bowl No1 7 spoons of aloe vera gel or neutral gel.

POUR INTO BOWL No2:

- Pour in the ingredients of phase B:

- 60 ml of witch hazel hydrosol / blueberry water. heat bowls No 1 and bowl No2 in a bain-marie for 10 minutes. pour the ingredients from bowl No1 into bowl No2.

- Using the spatula, mix the ingredients well to obtain a smooth, white and thick cream.

- Place the bowl in the bottom of cold water and continue to mix for a few minutes.

- Add the essential oils to the bowl glycerin and preservative / vitamin E.

- Transfer the cream to the jar / bottle.

- Use this cream up to 4 times / week.

24. CREAM ANTI AGING EVENING WITH SHEA BUTTER AND COCONUT

MATERIAL:

- 1 empty glass jar of 50 ml.
- 1 spatula.

INGREDIENTS:

- 25 g of Shea butter.
- 10 g of organic coconut vegetable oil.
- 1 large spoon of vegetable oil of hazelnut / grape seeds / carrots.
- 1 small spoonful of potato starch / cornstarch.
- 2 drops of vitamin E.

INSTRUCTIONS FOR USE:

- In the glass jar, pour the potato starch powder.
- Add the melted shea oil and coconut oil to the pot.
- Using the small spatula, mix all the ingredients well until a fluid and smooth cream is obtained.
- Close the jar and place it in 1 cool and dry place.
- Use this cream up to 4 times / week in the evening.

25. DAY CREAM FOR ALL SKIN

MATERIAL:

- 1 medium bowl.
- 1 empty 50ml glass jar.
- 1 spatula.

INGREDIENTS:

- 20g of melted beeswax.
- 20 ml of organic jojoba vegetable oil.
- 15 ml of cornflower / rose floral water.
- 7 drops of Giscard natural preservative / 4 drops of vitamin E.
- 2 drops of glycerin.

INSTRUCTIONS FOR USE:

- In 1 container, melt your beeswax in a bain-marie. take the container out of the bain-marie, pour the beeswax into the bowl.
- Add organic jojoba oil to the bowl.
- Add the floral water to the bowl, mix well with the spatula.
- Add vitamin E or the Cosgard preservative.
- Continue to mix the cream in the bowl until you obtain a fluid and smooth cream.
- Pour the cream into the glass cream jar. Close it well.
- You can store this cream in 1 cool place, but not in the refrigerator.

26. FIRMING CREAM FOR THE FACE AND NECK

MATERIAL:

- 1 small spatula.
- 1 empty 30ml (1 oz) glass cream jar.

INGREDIENTS:

- 30 g of deodorized lanolin.
- 5 drops of myrrh essential oil (it is an Ayurvedic oil).
- 5 drops of verbena essential oil.
- 5 drops of essential oil of geranium.

INSTRUCTIONS FOR USE:

- Pour the lanolin into the glass jar of cream.
- Add the essential oils
- Using the spatula, mix all the ingredients well, until a smooth and homogeneous cream is obtained.
- It is recommended to use this cream alternately with another treatment cream.

27. MOISTURIZING CREAM FOR ALL SKIN TYPES

INGREDIENTS:

- 1 medium size bowl.
- 1 spatula / mini mixer / mini whisk.
- 3 large spoons of organic vegetable oil of hemp / sweet almonds.
- 2 large spoons of shea butter / beeswax.
- 5 large spoons of witch hazel hydrosol / orange blossom.
- 1 teaspoon of organic aloe Vera gel.
- 5 drops of carrot / avocado essential oil.
- 3 drops of mandarin / grapefruit essential oil.
- 2 drops of hyaluronic acid.
- 1 drop of essential oil of Niaouli.
- 1/2 teaspoon of vitamin C powder.

DIRECTIONS:

- In the bowl, pour the vitamin C powder.
- Add the already melted shea butter / beeswax to the bowl.
- Mix well with the mini whisk to avoid lumps.
- Add the vegetable oil of hemp / sweet almonds, continue to mix.
- Add the 5 large spoons of hydrosol as well as the rest of the ingredients.
- Continue to mix well until you obtain a creamy and smooth cream.
- Transfer the cream to the jar. Keep the cream jar cool.

28. NOURISHING CREAM WITH CARROT AND ALMOND MILK

INGREDIENTS:

- 1 bottle / jar of 50ml.
- 1 small whisk / spatula / mini blender.
- 15 ml of mineral water.
- 30 ml of cornflower hydrosol / rose water.
- 1/2 teaspoon of organic glycerin.
- 1/2 teaspoon of carrot / avocado vegetable oil.
- 1/2 teaspoon of organic aloe vera powder / aloe Vera gel.
- 1 teaspoon of organic coconut milk powder.
- 1 drop of organic silicon.
- 2 drops of vitamin E.

DIRECTIONS FOR USE:

- In 1 medium bowl, dilute the aloe vera powder with mineral water.
- Add the organic coconut milk powder to the bowl and continue mixing well.
- Add the glycerin, continue to mix for 1 min.
- Add the cornflower hydrosol / rose water to the bowl.
- Add the rest of the ingredients.
- Continue to mix the cream well for 2 minutes until you obtain a creamy and smooth cream.
- Pour the cream into the jar, keep the cream in a cool place.

29. APRICOT GOOD GLOW DAY CREAM FOR ALL SKIN TYPES

INGREDIENTS:

- 2 medium size bowls.
- 1 small whisk.
- 1 syringe of 15 ml equal to 2 large spoons.
- 1 bottle of 100ml with pump / 1 glass jar of 100ml.

PHASE A:

- 15 ml of water oily macerate of carrots / avocado oil.
- 15 ml of vegetable oil of hazelnuts / apricot.
- 7 teaspoons of neutral gel. (Aloe Vera).

PHASE B:

- 60 ml of witch hazel hydrosol / blueberry water.

PHASE C:

- 15 drops of verbena / chamomile essential oil.
- 1 small spoonful of organic glycerin oil.
- 20 drops of cosgard preservative / 5 drops of vitamin E.

INSTRUCTIONS FOR USE:

- Put in the 1st bowl the ingredients of phase A (carrot macerate water, apricot vegetable oil / hazelnut oil, 7 teaspoons of neutral gel / aloe vera.

- In the 2nd bowl put the ingredients of phase B: 60 ml of witch hazel hydrosol / blueberry water.

- Heat phase A and phase B in a bain-marie.

- Carefully remove them from the heat 2 phase (A and B)

- Pour phase A into phase B. Using a spatula, mix all the ingredients well until a white, thick and homogeneous cream is obtained.

- Place the bowl in 1 in cold water and continue to mix for a few minutes to obtain a smooth and supple emulsion.

- Add the ingredients of phase C. (The essential oils, glycerin, preservative) to put the cream in a bottle or jar.

30. ANTI AGING FACE CREAM WITH NATURAL INGREDIENTS

- 25 g of Karate butter.
- 10 g of coconut vegetable oil.
- 1 large spoonful of organic hazelnut / grape seed / carrot vegetable oil.
- 1 small spoonful of potato starch / cornstarch.
- 2 drops of vitamin E.

INSTRUCTIONS FOR USE:

- In 1 glass jar, pour the potato starch / corn starch powder.
- Add the shea oils and coconut oil to the pot.
- Using a small spatula, mix well for a period of 1 min.
- Add the remaining ingredients with the spatula, Continue mixing well until a smooth cream is obtained.
- Close the jar, store the jar in a cool place (or in the fridge).
- Use this cream 4 times / week in the evening.

31. DAY CREAM FOR COMBINATION / OILY SKINS

INGREDIENTS:

- 1 glass jar of 50 ml.
- 25 ml of jojoba vegetable oil.
- 15 ml of cornflower / rose floral water.
- 7 drops of natural cosgard preservative.
- 1 drop of vitamin E / 1 drop of glycerin.
- 20g of beeswax.

DIRECTIONS:

- In 1 container, melt the beeswax in a Marie bath.
- Once the beeswax is melted, add the jojoba oil.
- Remove the container from the Marie bath.
- Add the floral water. Mix well.
- Add vitamin E.
- Add the Cosgard preservative.
- Continue stirring until you obtain a smooth and even cream.
- Pour the cream in the jar., Close the jar. Keep this cream in a cool place.

32. COUP D'ÉCLAT FACE CREAM RECIPE

MATERIAL:

- 1 glass of 30ml.
- 1 compress.

INGREDIENTS:

- 25 ml of organic almond / jojoba oil.
- 4 drops of rosewood essential oil.
- 3 drops of sandalwood / essential oil organic ginger.
- 5 drops of Frankincense essential/ oil carrot oil.

INSTRUCTIONS FOR USE:

- Pour all the ingredients into the bottle.
- Close the bottle tightly, shake the bottle energy for 1 minute.
- After removing make-up, use a few drops of this formula and massage the face and neck with your fingertips. Avoid the eye area.
- Keep this oil on your face overnight.
- In the morning, soak a compress in cornflower water / rosewater cleanse the skin.

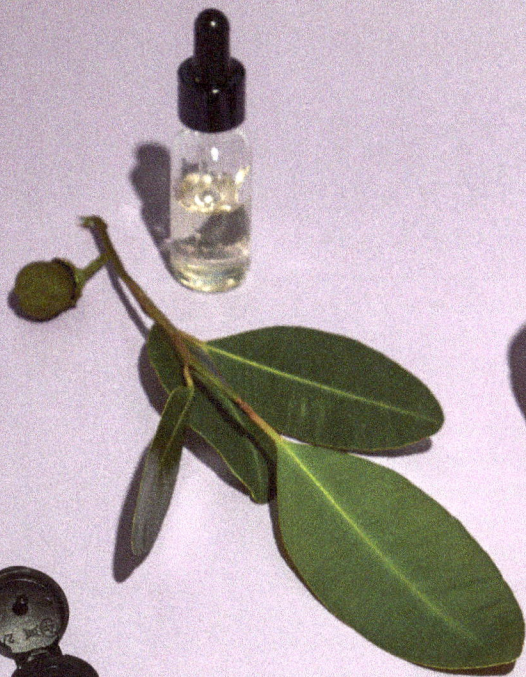

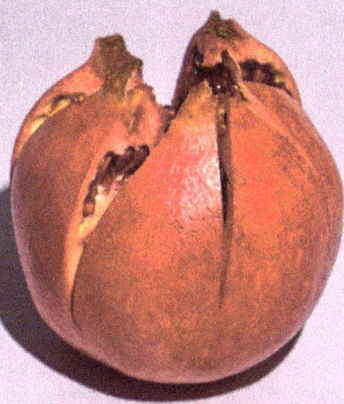

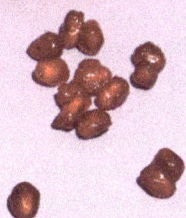

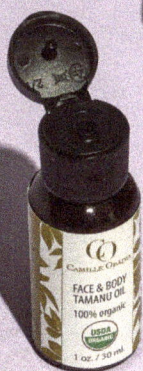

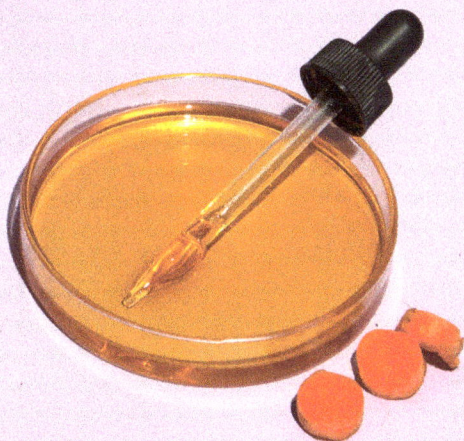

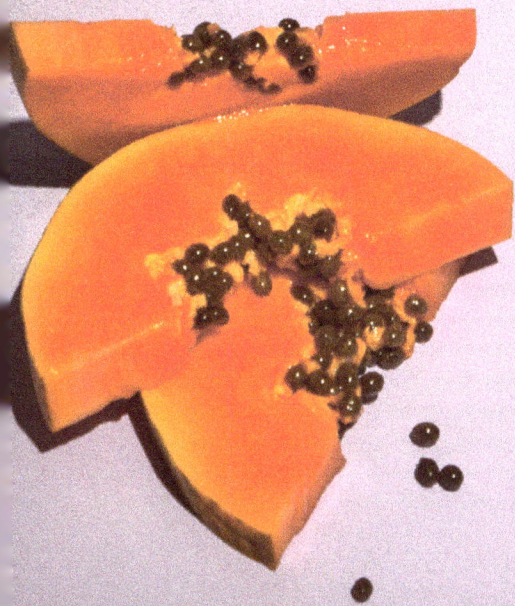

33. CREAM MOISTURIZING FOR COMBINATION SKIN

MATERIAL:

- 1 small blender.
- 1 spatula.
- 1 empty cream jar 50ml. glass.

INGREDIENTS:

- 1 large spoon of papaya fruit powder.
- 1 large spoon of grenadine juice (ready in organic bottle)—
- 2 drops of liquid zinc.
- 3 large spoons of floral water / hydrosol (homemade or purchased).
- 2 drops of liquid hyaluronic acid.
- 2 large spoons of organic jojoba vegetable oil.
- 2 drops of organic tamanu oil.
- 2 drops of carrot essential oil.

DIRECTIONS FOR USE:

- Pour all the ingredients into the small blender.
- Blend for 2 minutes.
- Pour the cream into the pot.
- Close the pot. Store the cream in 1 cool, dry place.
- Use this cream 3 times a week alternating with the cream conventional.

Anti Aging Serums and Anti Dark Circle Balms

---

34. ANTI WRINKLE SERUM WITH VITAMIN C

MATERIAL:

- 1 medium bowl.
- 1 spatula.
- 1 small brush.

INGREDIENTS:

- 1 glass bottle of 30 ml.
- 2 large spoons of cornflower / rose water.
- 3 teaspoons of vitamin C powder.
- 2 teaspoons of liquid glycerin.
- 1/2 teaspoon of oxygenating/ cream night cream.

DIRECTIONS:

- Pour vitamin C powder into the bowl and blueberry / rose water.
- Using the spatula, mix well until a fluid paste without obtained lumps is.
- Add the glycerin.
- Add the oxygenating cream or another day cream.
- Continue to mix to obtain 1 smooth fluid.
- Apply this serum on the face. Massage with your fingertips, focusing on wrinkles. Keep this serum on the skin overnight.
- Use this serum up to 4 times / week.

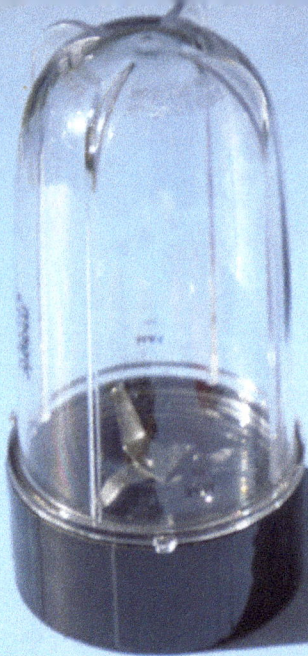

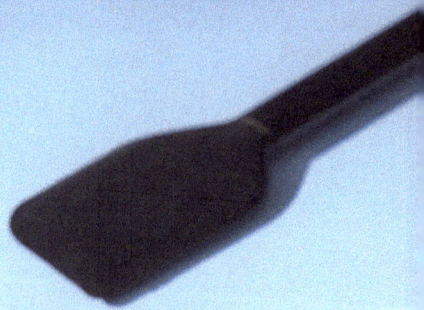

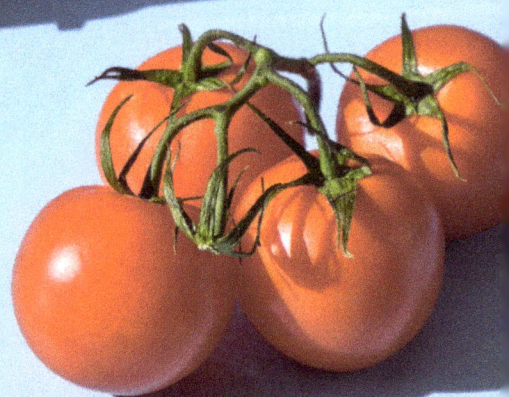

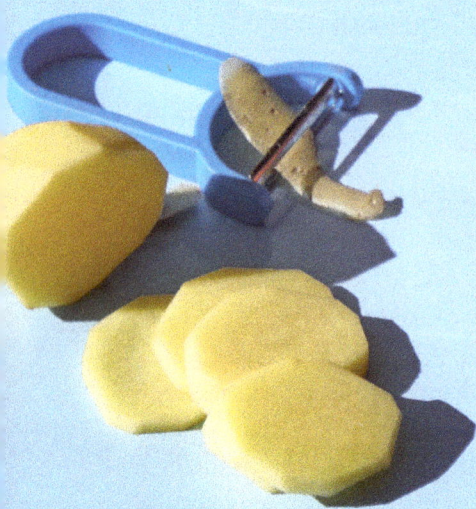

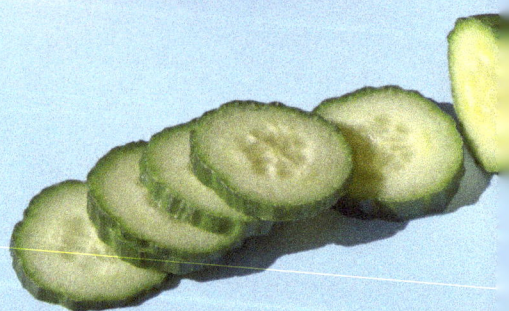

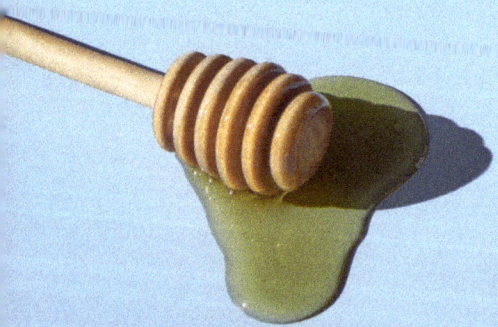

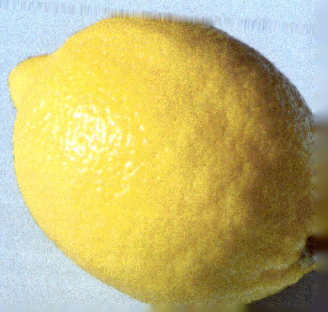

35. ANTI DARK CIRCLE CARE FOR THE EYES

MATERIAL:

- 1 mini blender.
- 1 medium bowl.
- 1 spatula.
- 2 large sterile compresses.

INGREDIENTS:

- 1/4 of fresh peeled tomatoes.
- 1 slice of peeled cucumber.
- 1 slice of peeled potato.
- 1 teaspoon of organic honey.
- 3 drops of fresh squeezed lemon.
- 2 large sterile compresses.

INSTRUCTIONS FOR USE:

- Pour all the ingredients into the blender.
- Blend for 2 minutes.
- Pour the contents of the blender into the bowl.
- Open 1 large compress, fold it in 4.
- Pour into the compress the amount of a teaspoon of this preparation.
- Fold the compress in 4 and place it under the eye. Do the same with the 2nd compress and place it under the 2nd eye.
- Keep these compresses for 10 minutes.
- Remove the compresses. Soak another cleanse compress in chamomile water,well under the eyes.
- Repeat this treatment up to 3 times / week.

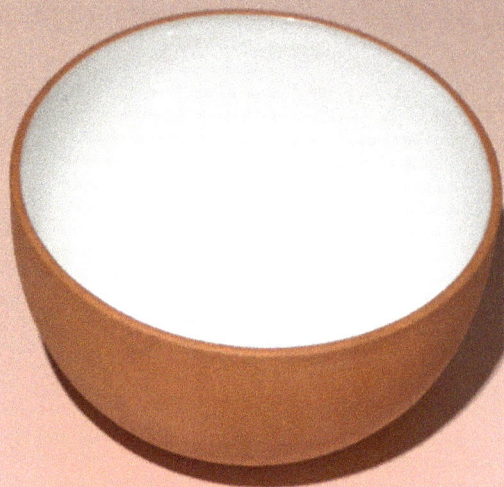

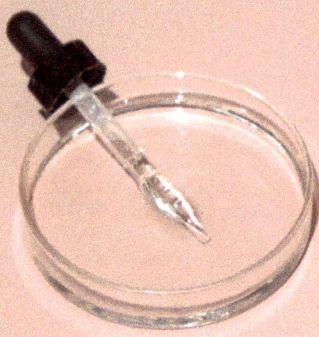

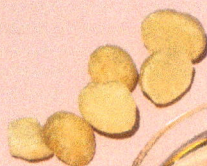

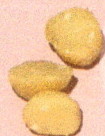

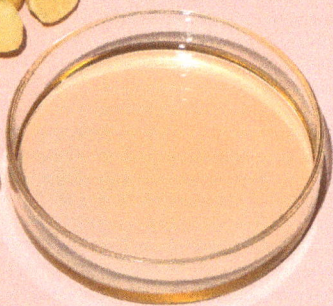

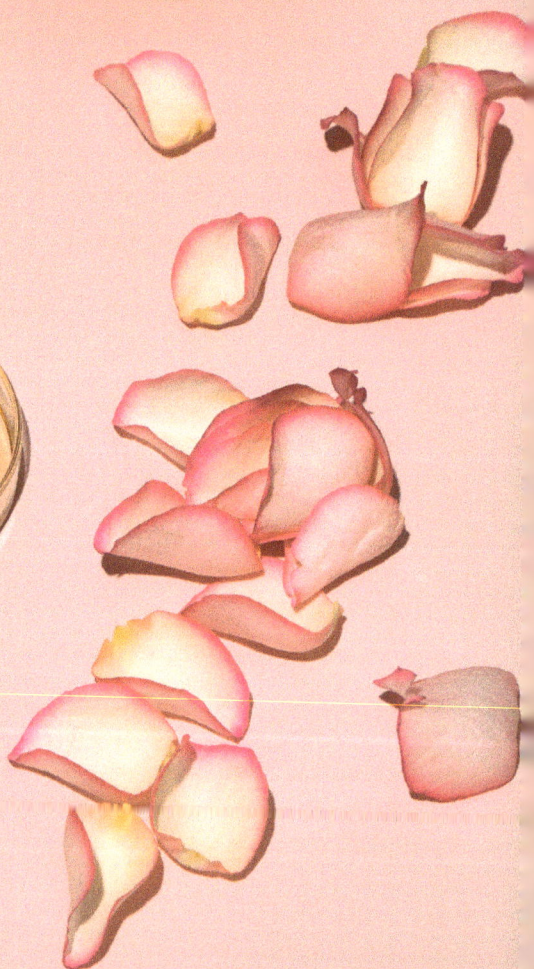

36. PERFUMED SERUM FOR THE FACE AND NECK

MATERIAL:

- 1 small dropper bottle of 15 ml.
- 1 medium bowl.
- 1 large sterile non-woven compress.

INGREDIENTS:

- 1 handful of fresh rose petals.
- 25 ml of macadamia vegetable oil / organic grape seed oil.
- 3 drops of rose essential oil.
- 2 drops of hyaluronic acid.
- 2 drops of vitamin E.

DIRECTIONS FOR USE:

- Place the rose petals in the bowl.
- Pour the vegetable macadamia oil over the rose petals.
- Cover the bowl, let macerate for 24 hours. filter the rose oil using the compress, collect the flavored oil.
- Pour this flavored oil into the bottle, add the rest of the ingredients.
- Close the bottle, shake it and let stand for 6 hours before use.
- 4 times / week, do not use this flavored oil in the evening.

37. CALMING EYE BEAUTY LOTION

MATERIAL:

- 3 large sterile, non-woven compresses.
- 1 Rapport.
- 1 small glass saucer.

INGREDIENTS :

- 1/2 cucumber.
- 2 drops of vitamin E.
- 2 drops of organic chamomile essential oil.
- 2 drops of organic aloe Vera gel.

DIRECTIONS:

- Peel the 1/2 cucumber. Grate it.
- Open 1 compress, place the grated cucumber in it.
- Close the compress. Squeeze the compress to collect the juice from the cucumber.
- Collect the juice of the cucumber in the small saucer. add vitamin E, 2 drops of Aloe Vera and to the small saucer the 2 drops of chamomile essential oil.
- Mix the ingredients and soak the 2 compresses.
- Place the compresses on your eyes for a period of 10 minutes.
- Repeat this treatment up to 2 times / week.

38. SERUM BEAUTY ANTI WRINKLE VITAMIN C

INGREDIENTS:

- 1 small bowl.
- 1 spatula + 1 brush.
- 2 large spoons of rose / cornflower water.
- 3 teaspoons of vitamin C powder.
- 2 teaspoons of glycerin (oil).
- 1/2 teaspoon of oxygenating cream.

DIRECTIONS:

- In the small bowl, mix the vitamin C powder with rose / blueberry water.
- Dilute the vitamin C powder well until you obtain a cream without lumps.
- Add glycerin.
- Add the oxygenating cream. Continue to mix to obtain a fluid and smooth cream.
- Apply this serum to the face, focusing on wrinkles.
- Use this treatment up to 4X / week, evening wheat.

39. RECIPE FOR DARK CIRCLES UNDER EYES

INGREDIENTS :

- 1 blender.
- 1/4 peeled fresh tomato.
- 1 slice of peeled cucumber.
- 1 slice of peeled potato.
- 1 teaspoon of organic honey.
- 3 drops of fresh squeezed lemon.
- 2 compresses.

INSTRUCTIONS FOR USE:

- In the blender, combine all the ingredients.
- Mix for 2 minutes.
- Pour the contents of the blender into 1 small bowl.
- Open a compress, pour in the compress 1 teaspoon of this preparation. Fold the compress in 4 and place the compress under the eyes. Do the same with the compress and place it under the 2nd eye.
- Keep the compress for 10 minutes, remove, then soak another compress in blueberry water, clean the remaining ingredients.
- Repeat this treatment up to 3X / week.

40. BALM FOR A ZEN AND CONTINUOUS SLEEP RECIPE

INGREDIENTS :

- 1 1/2 large spoon of beeswax / shea butter.
- 2 large spoons of organic linseed / macadamia vegetable oil.
- 10 drops of chamomile essential oil.
- 5 drops of lavender essential oil.
- 3 drops of basil essential oil
- 2 drops of organic ginger essential oil.

DIRECTIONS:

- In 1 medium bowl, pour beeswax / shea butter.
- Place the bowl in a Bain Marie, let the beeswax / shea butter melt.–Add flaxseed / macadamia vegetable oil. Mix well with the spatula.
- Remove the bowl from the Marie bath.
- Add essential oils. Continue to mix well for 2 minutes.
- Pour the preparation into 1 glass jar.
- Close the jar and store in 1 cool place.
- Every evening, use this balm in massage on the temples, the inside of the wrists and in the hollow of the neck.

41. PLANT MOISTURIZING LIP BALM

INGREDIENTS:

- 1 medium bowl.
- 2 teaspoons of hazelnut vegetable oil / mango vegetable oil.
- 1/2 teaspoon of beeswax.
- 1 teaspoon of acacia honey.
- 4 drops of macadamia vegetable oil.
- 1 drop of vitamin E.

INSTRUCTIONS FOR USE:

- Pour the vegetable oils into the bowl.
- Place the bowl in the Marie bath. Mix the ingredients well in the bowl.
- Add the rest of the ingredients.
- Remove the bowl from the Marie bath.
- Let cool. Pour the preparation into the jar / bottle.
- Use this balm for your lips several times a day.

42. DECONGESTING BALM FOR THE EYE CONTOUR

INGREDIENTS:

- 1 bottle / jar of 100ml.
- 1 small spatula.
- 1/2 teaspoonful of Nescafé powder.
- 1 teaspoon of beeswax.
- 40 g of mango / coconut butter.
- 1 large spoonful of jojoba vegetable oil.
- 6 drops of Arnica essential oil.
- 4 drops of vitamin E.
- 4 drops of Helichrysum essential oil.

INSTRUCTIONS FOR USE

- Pour the beeswax, mango butter, coconut butter into the bowl.
- Place the bowl in the Marie bath. Using the spatula, mix well.
- Add the Nescafe powder, continue to mix.
- Add jojoba vegetable oil, arenicolid essential, Helichrysum essential, vitamin E.
- Mix well. Take the bowl out of the Marie bath. Let cool.
- Pour the preparation into the jar / bottle.
- Every evening, use this balm for the eye area.

43. ANTI WRINKLE FACE OIL RECIPE

INGREDIENTS:

- 1 glass bottle of 20 ml.
- 18 ml of sweet almond oil.
- 4 drops of patchouli essential oil.
- 2 drops of lime essential oil.
- 4 drops of rose essential oil.
- 5 drops of carrot essential oil.

INSTRUCTIONS FOR USE:

- Pour all the ingredients into the glass bottle.
- Close the bottle well, shake it for 1 minute.
- On well cleansed skin, massage with this oil (fingertips) for a period of 1-2 minutes. Avoid the eye area.
- Keep for a few hours.
- Repeat this treatment 4 times / week.

44. ANTI AGING SERUM WITH GRAPE SEEDS

MATERIAL:

- 1 bottle of 100 ml.

INGREDIENTS:

- 30 ml of organic grape seed oil.
- 30 ml of organic linseed oil.
- 30 ml of macadamia oil.
- 10 ml of organic glycerin oil.
- 5 drops of calendula essential oil.
- 5 drops of lavender essential oil.
- 10 drops of cornflower essential oil.

INSTRUCTIONS FOR USE:

- Pour the oils: flax, grape seeds into the bottle.
- Close the bottle, shake it for 1 minute.
- Open the bottle, add the oils essential. Close the bottle.
- Shake the bottle for 1 minute. use 5-6 drops on the skin in a circular massage.

45. SOOTHING ANTI REDNESS FACE OIL

MATERIAL:

- 1 bottle of 30 ml in dropper glass.

INGREDIENTS:

- 27 ml of Calendula oil / organic linseed oil.
- 20 drops of lavender essential oil.
- 2 drops of carrot essential oil.
- 10 drops of organic tamanu oil.
- 5 drops of organic Aloe Vera gel.

INSTRUCTIONS FOR USE:

- Pour all the ingredients into the bottle.
- Close the bottle. Shake the bottle for 2 minutes.
- Before each use of this oil, shake the bottle well.
- Use a few drops of this oil on parts of the skin irritated and after sunburn.
- Store away from light.

Face Masks

46. DETOXIFYING MASK

INGREDIENTS:

- 1 teaspoon of fresh brewer's yeast granules.
- 2 small spoons of lukewarm fresh milk.
- 1 small spoonful of honey.
- 1/4 of fresh yogurt.
- 1 small bowl.
- 1 spatula.

DIRECTIONS:

- In 1 glass, mix the brewer's yeast and the milk, (let stand in 1 warm place) for 20 minutes.
- In 1 bowl, pour the brewer's yeast (already diluted in the milk)
- Add the 1/4 yogurt.
- Using the spatula, mix well until a smooth paste is obtained.
- With the spatula, spread the paste on the face.
- Keep the mask on for 15 minutes. Rinse it off with lukewarm water. Dry the skin. Using a compress soaked in lime blossom water, wash off the rest of the mask.

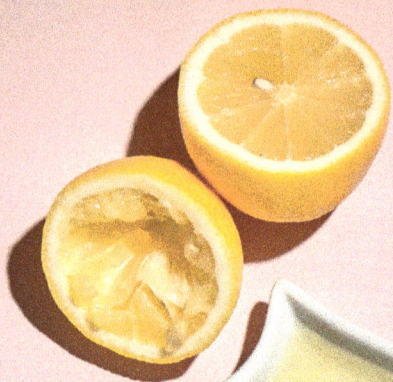

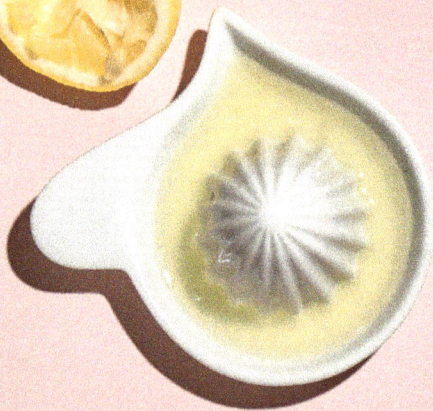

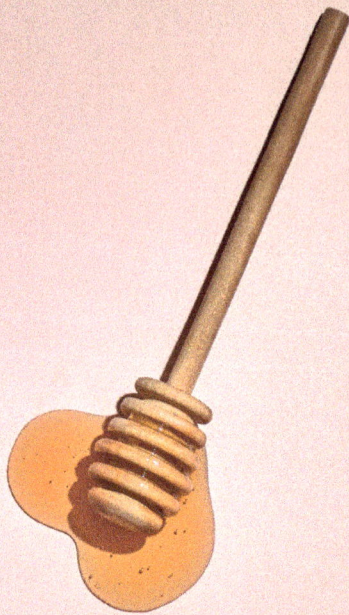

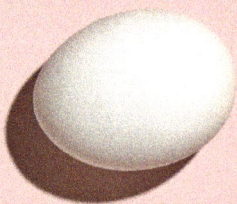

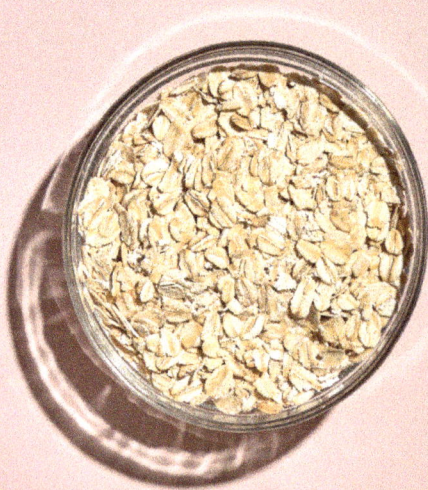

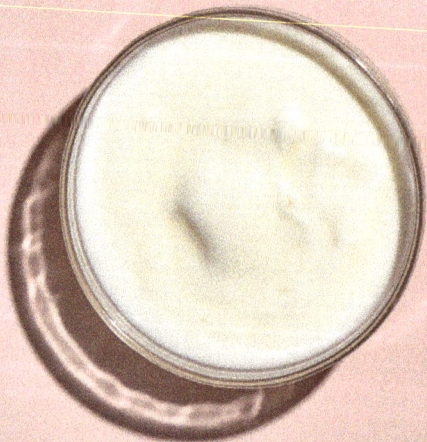

47. OATMEAL EXFOLIATING MASK RECIPE

INGREDIENTS:

- 1/2 cup hot water.
- 3 large spoons of oatmeal.
- 2 teaspoons of honey.
- 1 large spoonful of yogurt
- 1 egg white.
- 4 drops of fresh squeezed lemon.
- 2 drops of organic glycerin.

DIRECTIONS:

- In 1 small saucepan, heat 1/2 large cup of water.
- Carefully pour warm water into 1 medium bowl.
- Add the 3 large spoons of oatmeal to the bowl.
- Using a spatula, mix well for 2 minutes.
- Add the rest of the ingredients. Mix well until obtained a homogeneous paste is.
- Using the spatula, cover the face with this mask. Keep for 15 minutes.
- Rinse off with lukewarm water.
- Soak 1 compress in rose water / witch hazel, Clean the rest of the mask.

48. BEAUTY FACE MASK TO ILLUMINATE THE COMPLEXION AND TIGHTEN THE PORES

INGREDIENTS:

- 1 blender.
- 2 slices of peeled cucumber.
- 1 large tablespoon of honey.
- 1 fresh carrot peeled and grated.
- 1/2 Greek yogurt.
- 1 teaspoon of organic avocado oil.
- 1 spatula.
- 1 1 small bowl.

INSTRUCTIONS FOR USE:

- Gather all the ingredients in the blender.
- Mix well for 3 minutes.
- Pour the preparation into the bowl.
- Using the spatula, spread this mask in a thick layer on the face.
- Break time 20-25 minutes. Rinse it off with lukewarm water.
- Using a compress soaked in aloe vera water, remove the rest of the mask.
- This mask is recommended 1X / week.

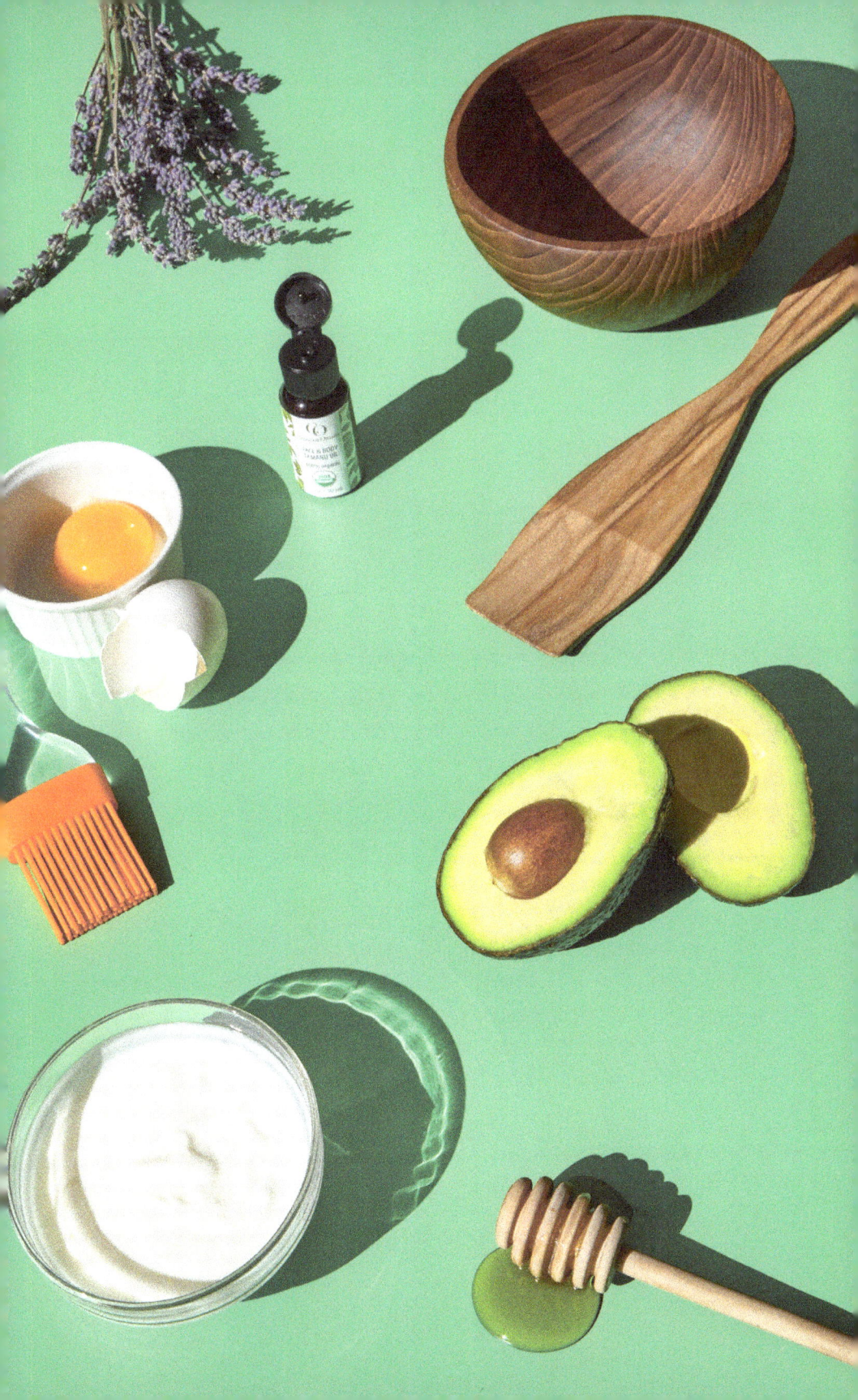

49. FRESH MASK FOR ALL SKIN

MATERIAL:

- 1 medium bowl.
- 1 spatula.
- 1 brush.

INGREDIENTS:

- 10 drops of organic tamanu oil.
- 2 drops of organic lavender essential oil.
- 1: 4 fresh squeezed lemon juice.
- 2 large spoons of creme fraiche.
- 1 egg yolk.
- 1 teaspoon of honey.
- 1/2 spoon of crushed fresh avocado.

INSTRUCTIONS FOR USE:

- Pour all the ingredients into the bowl.
- Using the spatula, mix all the ingredients well until a smooth cream is obtained.
- Using the brush, spread the mask in a thick layer on the face and neck.
- Keep the mask on for 15-20 minutes.
- Rinse off with lukewarm water.
- Soak a compress in water
- Aloe Vera and wash off the rest of the mask. Finish with a moisturizer.

50. MASK FOR DRY HAIR RECIPE

INGREDIENTS:

- 1 medium bowl.
- 1 spatula and 1 fork.
- 1 egg yolk.
- 5 drops of castor oil / organic argan oil.
- 1/2 fresh banana.
- 1 1/2 of organic acacia honey.
- 3 spoons of hazelnut / almond oil.

DIRECTIONS:

- In the bowl, mash the banana with the fork.
- Add the egg yolk to the bowl, mix well using the mini whisk / spatula.
- Add organic acacia honey, continue mixing.
- Add the hazelnut / almond oil.
- Add the argan / castor oil while continuing to mix, until a smooth and creamy paste is obtained.
- Transfer the mask to 1 jar, close the jar and store in 1 cool place.

51. FACE MASK TO BRIGHTEN BROWN SPOTS

INGREDIENTS:

- 2 large spoons of milk powder.
- 2 small spoons of brown sugar.
- 1 teaspoon of organic hemp oil or avocado oil.
- 1 tomato cut in 2.
- 2 drops of tamanu oil or grapefruit essential oil.

MATERIAL:

- 1 medium bowl.
- 1 spatula.

DIRECTIONS:

- Pour in the sugar, powdered milk and tamanu oil or essential oil grapefruit.
- Using the spatula, mix the ingredients well.
- Use the 1/2 tomato, dip it in the preparation and with this 1/2 tomato
- Massage the parts of the skin for 2 minutes, insisting on brown spots. Rinse it off with lukewarm water.
- Soak a compress with cornflower water / rose water and wash off the rest of the mask.
- Use an unscented moisturizer.
- You can repeat this mask up to 2 times / week.

52. MASK FOR OILY SKIN

INGREDIENTS:

- 4 large spoons of calcium clay powder.
- 2 large spoons of organic cider vinegar.
- 3 large spoons of organic aloe vera water.
- 2 large spoons of which hazel / hydrosol floral water.
- 6 drops of grapefruit / peppermint / sage essential oil.

MATERIAL:

- 1 medium bowl.
- 1 spatula.
- 1 brush.
- 1 compress.

INSTRUCTIONS FOR USE:

- Pour all the ingredients into the bowl.
- Using the spatula, mix all the ingredients well until you obtain a smooth and homogeneous cream.
- Using the brush, spread the mask only on the face.
- Keep the mask on for 15-20 minutes.
- Rinse off the mask with lukewarm water.
- Soak the compress with rosemary or orange blossom / hydrosol floral water.
- You can repeat this mask 2-3 times / week.

53. MASK FOR DRY HAIR WITH ALMOND OIL

INGREDIENTS:

- 5 large spoons of organic almond oil.
- 1 egg yolk.
- 1 small spoonful of honey.
- 10 drops of fresh squeezed lemon juice.
- 1 teaspoon of organic cider vinegar.
- 4 drops of organic tamanu oil or hemp oil.

MATERIAL:

- 1 spatula.
- 1 medium bowl.
- 1 plastic shower cap.
- 1 shampoo for dry hair.

DIRECTIONS:

- Pour all the ingredients into the bowl.
- Using the spatula, mix all the ingredients well until obtained a homogeneous and smooth cream.
- Apply this mask along the length of your slightly damp hair.
- Cover your hair with 1 plastic cap and keep this mask for a period of 20 minutes.
- Wash your hair with shampoo.

54. FRESH VEGETABLES MASK FOR ALL SKIN

INGREDIENTS:

- 1 large pumpkin slice.
- 1/4 fresh avocado.
- 2 small slices of fresh ginger.
- 2 spoons of fresh cream.
- 5 drops of organic almond oil.
- 5 drops of organic tamanu oil.
- 5 drops of lavender essential oil.
- 5 spoons of coconut powder.

MATERIAL:

- 1 blender
- 1 medium bowl.
- 1 brush

INSTRUCTIONS FOR USE:

- Put all of the ingredients into the blender and mix for 2 minutes.
- Put this mask into a medium bowl.
- Clean your face and neck.
- Using the brush cover your face and neck with the mask (avoid eye area).
- Leave this mask on for 15 minuets then carefully rinse your face and neck with lukewarm water.

55. ANTI AGING ARGAN OIL MASK

INGREDIENTS:

- 3 large spoons of white clay powder.
- 1 large spoon of organic argan oil.
- 1/4 glass of rose water or witch hazel hydrosol water.
- 6 drops of cornflower or orange blossom essential oil.

MATERIAL:

- 1 medium bowl.
- 1 spatula.
- 1 compress.

INSTRUCTIONS FOR USE:

- Pour all the ingredients into the bowl.
- Using the spatula, mix all the ingredients well until obtained a smooth paste without lumps is.
- Using the spatula, apply the mask, in a thick layer, on the face and neck (avoid the eye area).
- Keep the mask on for 15-20 minutes—Rinse the mask off with lukewarm water.
- Soak the compress in blueberry water or witch hazel water, thoroughly clean the rest of the mask.

56. MASK FOR ALL SKIN

INGREDIENTS:

- 2 large spoons of rice flour.
- 1 teaspoon of organic aloe vera gel.
- 2 drops of organic tamanu oil.
- 2 drops of essential oil of cornflower or rose.
- 10 drops of liquid glycerin.
- 1/2 cup of lukewarm chamomile water.

MATERIAL:

- 1 medium bowl.
- 1 spatula.
- 1 brush.
- 1 compress.

INSTRUCTIONS FOR USE:

- Pour all the ingredients into the bowl.
- Using the spatula, mix all the ingredients well until a smooth and homogeneous paste is obtained.
- Using the brush, spread the mask over the face and neck, and around the eye area.
- Keep the mask on for 20 minutes. Rinse it off with lukewarm water.
- Soak 1 compress in chamomile water and clean the rest of the mask.
- Use a cream rich in vitamin E.

57. ANTI AGING ROSE MUSK MASK: ROSEHIP

INGREDIENTS:

- 30 ml of vegetable oil or sesame oil.
- 5 ml of avocado vegetable oil.
- 15 drops of verbena essential oil.
- 2 capsules of vitamin E.

MATERIAL:

- 1 medium bowl.
- 1 spatula.
- 1 brush.
- 1 compress.

INSTRUCTIONS FOR USE:

- Pour all the ingredients into the bowl.
- With the spatula, mix all the ingredients well.
- Apply the mask with your fingertips and massage with your face for 3 minutes. Using the brush, spread the rest of the mask on the skin.
- Keep the mask for 15 minutes, remove the mask using the compress soaked in cornflower or rose water.

58. ANTI WRINKLE MASK WITH GUMBO VEGETABLE (GAMBA)

INGREDIENTS:

- 4 fresh GOMBO, without the stems.
- 1 egg white.
- 3 drops of carrot essential oil.
- 5 drops of fresh squeezed lemon juice.
- 1 teaspoon of Aloe Vera gel.
- 1 vitamin E capsule.

MATERIALS:

- 1 mini blender.
- 1 medium bowl.
- 1 spatula.
- 1 brush.
- 1 compress.

INSTRUCTIONS FOR USE:

- Pour the GOMBO vegetable into the blender, (first cut the vegetable into strips).
- Add the egg white to the blender. Blend for 1 minute.
- Add the drops of carrot essential oil to the blender. Mix for a period of 2 minutes.
- Pour everything into the bowl. Add to it:
- Lemon, vitamin E, and Aloe Vera. Mix well with the spatula.
- Using the brush, spread the mask over the face. Keep the mask on for 15 minutes.
- Rinse off the mask with lukewarm water.
- Soak a compress with verbena water or lime blossom water.
- Finish with an anti-aging cream.

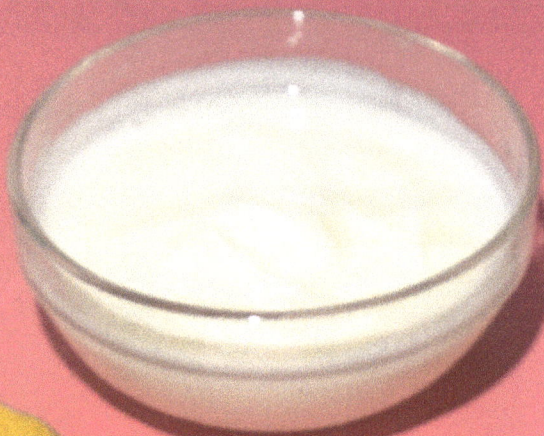

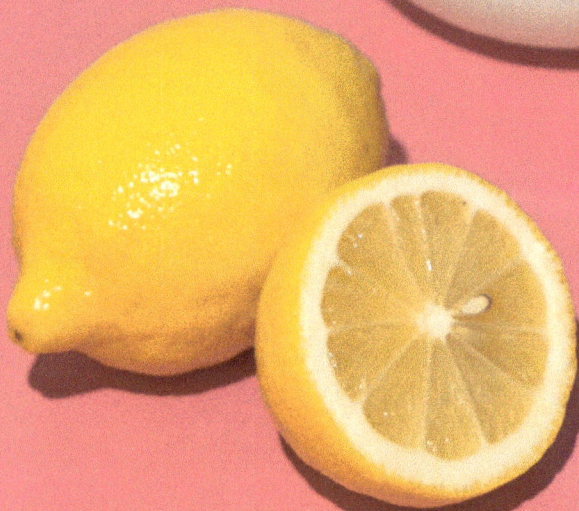

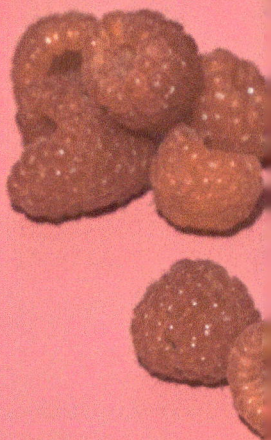

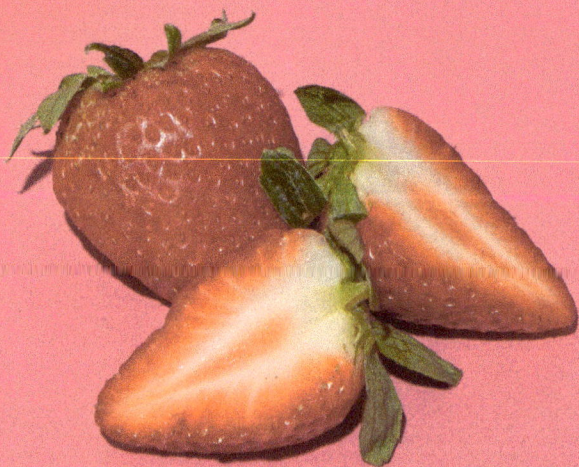

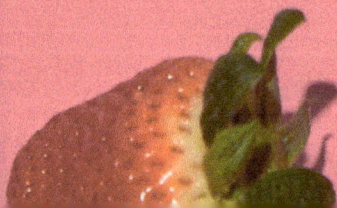

59. RED FRUIT MASK

INGREDIENTS:

- Juice of 1 fresh lemon.
- 80 grams of fresh strawberries.
- 80 grams of fresh raspberries.
- 3 small spoons of crème fraiche.

MATERIAL:

- 1 small mixer / blender.
- 1 spatula.
- 1 medium bowl.

INSTRUCTIONS FOR USE:

- Pour all the ingredients into the blender. Blend for 2 minutes.
- Pour the mask into the bowl.
- Using the spatula, spread this mask in a thick layer all over the face, avoiding the eye area.
- Keep the mask on for 20 minutes.
- Rinse the mask off with lukewarm water.
- Soak 1 compress in a verbena tonic, clean the rest of the mask.
- Use 1 moisturizer for normal skin.

60. COFFEE MASK FOR ALL SKIN

INGREDIENTS:

- 3 large spoons of ground coffee.
- 1/4 glass of lukewarm milk.
- 7 drops of organic rose essential oil.
- 1 capsule of vitamin E.
- 5 drops of essential oil of cinnamon.

MATERIAL:

- 1 medium bowl.
- 1 spatula.

INSTRUCTIONS FOR USE:

- Pour all the ingredients into the bowl.
- Using the spatula, mix all the ingredients well until a smooth and creamy paste is obtained.
- Using the spatula, spread the mask over the face.
- Keep the mask on for 15 minutes.
- Rinse off the mask with lukewarm water.
- Soak the compress in an organic chamomile / linden tonic.
- Finish with a moisturizer for all skin types.

61. BRIGHTENING AND ANTI-SPOTS MASK WITH POTATOES

INGREDIENTS:

- 1 medium potato.
- 2 teaspoons of fresh lemon juice.

MATERIAL:

- 1 medium bowl.
- 1 spatula.
- 1 brush.
- 1 compress.

INSTRUCTIONS FOR USE:

- Wash the potato well. Dry it.
- Grate the potato (with its peel).
- Open a compress, add the already grated potato and extract the potato juices.
- Pour the potato juice into the bowl.
- Add 2 teaspoons of fresh lemon. using the spatula, mix all the ingredients in the bowl until you obtain a smooth and fluid cream.
- Using the brush, spread the mask over the face (avoid the eye area).
- Keep the mask on for 15 minutes, rinse with lukewarm water.
- Repeat this mask 2 times / week. It is excellent for brightening the complexion and dark spots.

62. PURIFYING CLAY MASK, FOR OILY AND COMBINATION SKIN

INGREDIENTS:

- 1 1/2 large spoon of white clay powder.
- 10 drops of organic tamanu oil.
- 3 large spoons of mineral water.
- 2 drops of essential oil of geranium or rosemary.
- 4 drops of vitamin E = 2 capsules.

MATERIAL:

- 1 medium bowl.
- 1 spatula.
- 1 brush. compress.

INSTRUCTIONS FOR USE:

- Pour all the ingredients into the bowl.
- Using the spatula, mix the ingredients until you obtain a smooth cream.
- Using the brush, spread the mask in a thick layer over the entire face and neck, avoiding the eye area.
- Keep the mask on for 20 minutes.
- Rinse off with lukewarm water.
- Soak a compress in the witch hazel tonic, Clean the rest of the mask.
- Finish with 1 short massage with 2 drops of vitamin E.

63. PURIFYING MASK FOR COMBINATION AND OILY SKIN

INGREDIENTS:

- 3 large spoons of oatmeal.
- 5 large spoons of verbena or mineral water.
- 1 teaspoon of organic aloe Vera gel.
- 1 teaspoon of organic cider vinegar.
- 4 drops of essential oil of ginger.

MATERIAL:

- 1 medium bowl.
- 1 spatula. sterile compress.

INSTRUCTIONS FOR USE:

- Pour all the ingredients into the bowl.
- Using the spatula, mix well until a smooth paste is obtained.
- With the spatula, spread the mask in a thick layer all over the face (Avoid the eye area).
- Keep the mask on for 20 minutes.
- Rinse the mask off with lukewarm water.
- Soak a compress in a witch hazel tonic and remove the rest of the mask from the skin.

64. PURIFYING MASK FOR COMBINATION SKIN

INGREDIENTS:

- 30g of brewer's yeast.
- 2 large spoons of organic honey.
- 1/2 Greek yogurt.
- 2 drops of organic lemon essential oil.
- 2 large spoons of organic Aloe Vera gel.
- 4 drops of grapefruit essential oil.

MATERIALS:

- 1 medium bowl.
- 1 spatula.
- 1 brush.

INSTRUCTIONS FOR USE:

- In the bowl, dilute and mix the brewer's yeast and the Greek yogurt.
- Pour the remaining ingredients into the bowl.
- Using the spatula, mix all the ingredients until you obtain a smooth cream without lumps.
- Using the brush, spread the mask over the face (avoid eye area) and neck in a thick layer.
- Keep the mask on for 25 minutes.
- Rinse off the mask with lukewarm water.
- Remove the rest of the mask with a compress soaked in lime water.

65. GELATIN FACE PEELING

MATERIAL:

- 1 medium bowl.
- 1 spatula.
- 1 brush.
- 1 scissors.

INGREDIENTS:

- 1 gelatin sheet.
- 2 drops of organic silicon.
- 1/2 teaspoon of active elastin powder / Aloe Vera gel.
- 1/4 glass of warm soy milk.
- 2 drops of rose / chamomile essential oil.

INSTRUCTIONS FOR USE:

- Using scissors above the bowl, cut them into small pieces collagen sheet.
- In the bowl, pour the warm soy milk and mix with the spatula until the collagen sheet has completely melted.
- Add the remaining ingredients to the bowl.
- Using the spatula mix for 1 minute.
- Using the brush, spread this peel on your skin. Break time
- 12 minutes.
- Rinse off with lukewarm water. Pat your skin dry and use moisturizer.
- Repeat this peeling mask twice a week.

66. MASK FOR DILATED PORES ANTI COMEDONES

MATERIAL:

- 1 small bowl.
- 1 spatula.
- 1 hot damp towel.
- 1 brush.

INGREDIENTS:

- 1 egg white.
- 1 small spoon of vegetable oil of apricot kernels / organic hemp oil.
- 1 small teaspoon of baking soda powder.
- 1 pinch of cinnamon powder.

INSTRUCTIONS FOR USE:

- Wet the towel, wring it out, then place the towel in the microwave for 35 seconds. take the towel out of the microwave. Open the towel, then cover the face with this warm towel for 3 minutes. in the small bowl, pour all the ingredients, mix well for 1 minute.
- Remove the towel, using the brush, spread this mask on the face, avoiding the eye area.
- Break time: 20 minutes.
- Rinse off with lukewarm water. Then, do not use a cream containing zinc and vitamin C.

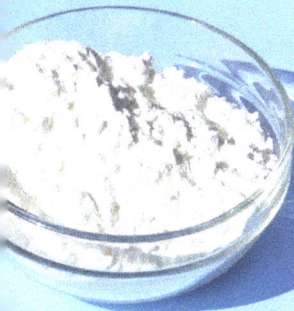

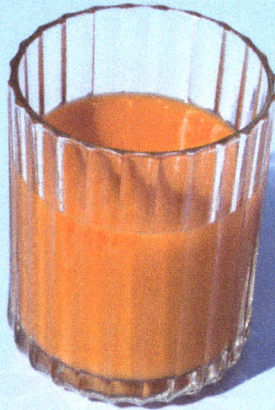

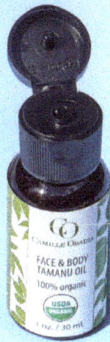

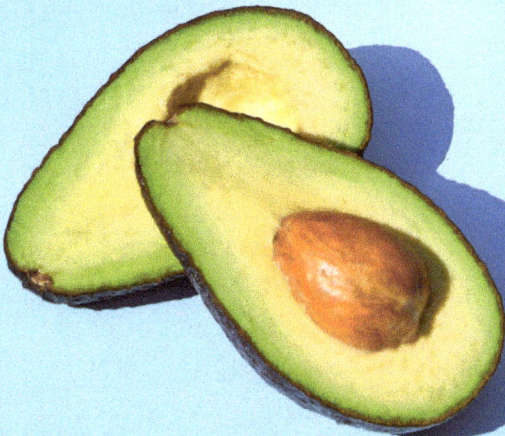

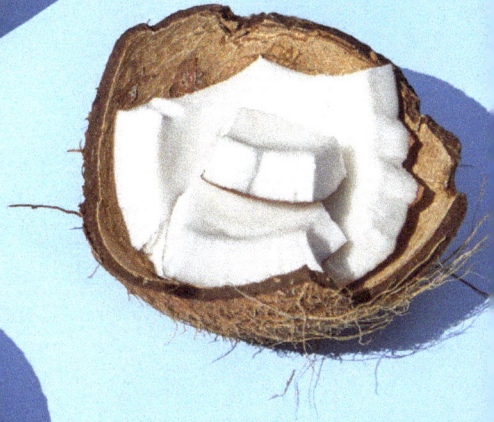

67. MOISTURIZING LIFT EFFECT MASK

MATERIAL:

- 1 medium bowl.
- 1 spatula.
- 1 small saucepan.

INGREDIENTS:

- 4 large spoons of fresh carrot juice.
- 1 large spoon of organic coconut oil.
- 1 teaspoon of avocado vegetable oil organic macadamia.
- 10 drops of organic tamanu oil.
- 1 1/2 large spoon of corn flour.
- 1 teaspoon of organic honey.

DIRECTIONS:

- In the bowl, dilute the corn flour with 1/2 glass of water.
- In the small saucepan, carefully pour 100 ml of boiling water. Add the pan already diluted corn flour too.
- Keep the saucepan on low heat while continuing to mix with the spatula until a thick paste is obtained.
- Let cool. Add the carrot juice, tamanu oil, coconut oil, honey, and macadamia / avocado oil.
- Using the spatula, spread the mask in a thick layer over the entire face.
- Keep the mask on for 20 minutes, rinse off with lukewarm water.
- The rest of the mask can be stored in the refrigerator.
- Repeat this mask 2 days in a row.

68. CURCUMA MASK

INGREDIENTS:

- 1 medium bowl.
- 1 spatula / mini whisk.
- 2 teaspoons of rice powder.
- 1/2 teaspoon of curcuma powder.
- 1 small spoon of vegetable oil of hemp / flax / sweet almonds.
- 2 drops of organic liquid zinc. drops of ginger / grapefruit essential oil.
- 1 large spoonful of organic soy milk.

INSTRUCTIONS FOR USE:

- In the bowl, pour the rice powder, the curcumin powder.
- Add vegetable oil to the bowl and mix well for 1 minute.
- Add the soy milk to the bowl, continue to mix for 1 minute, and until a smooth paste without lumps is obtained.
- Using the spatula, cover the blackhead parts of the skin.
- Keep the mask on for 30 minutes.
- Rinse off the mask with water.
- Soak 1 compress in cornflower tonic / witch hazel water.

69. BEAUTY MASK WITH ARGAN OIL—ANTI AGING

INGREDIENTS:

- 3 large spoons of white clay powder.
- 1 large spoon of organic argan oil.
- 1/4 glass of rose water.
- 3 drops of carrot essential oil / rose essential oil.

DIRECTIONS:

- In 1 medium bowl, assemble all ingredients.
- Using a spatula, mix all the ingredients well until you obtain a smooth and creamy paste.
- Using the spatula, apply the mask in a thick layer (avoid the eye area).
- Keep the mask on for 15-20 minutes.
- Rince with lukewarm water. Using a compress soaked in cornflower floral water/rose water, clean the rest of the mask.

70. MASK FOR DRY HAIR WITH SWEET ALMOND OIL

INGREDIENTS:

- 5 large spoons of organic sweet almond oil.
- 1 egg yolk.
- 1 small spoonful of honey.
- 10 drops of fresh lemon juice.
- 1 teaspoon of apple cider vinegar.

DIRECTIONS:

- In 1 medium bowl, mix all ingredients.
- Using a spatula, mix well until a smooth cream is obtained. on slightly damp hair, apply the mask along the length of the hair.
- Keep the mask on the hair for 15-20 minutes.
- Wash your hair with 1 mild hair shampoo.

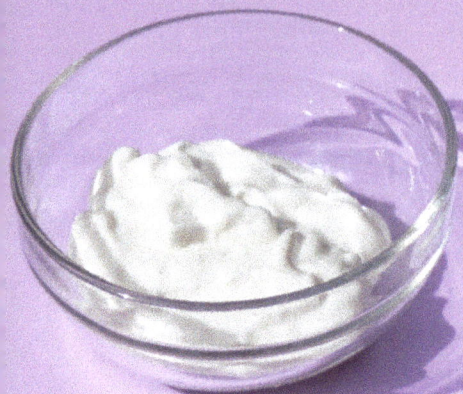

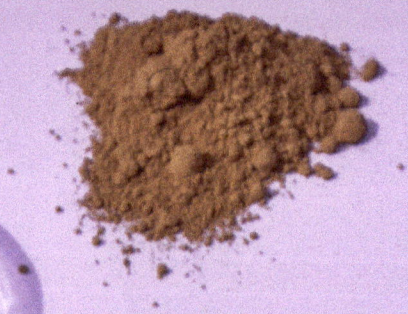

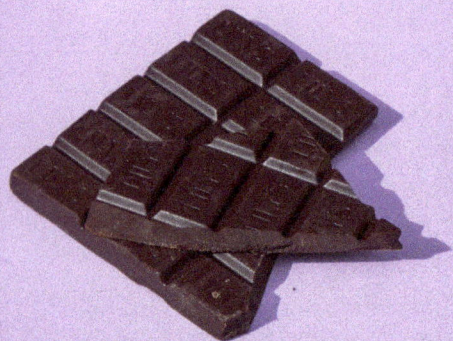

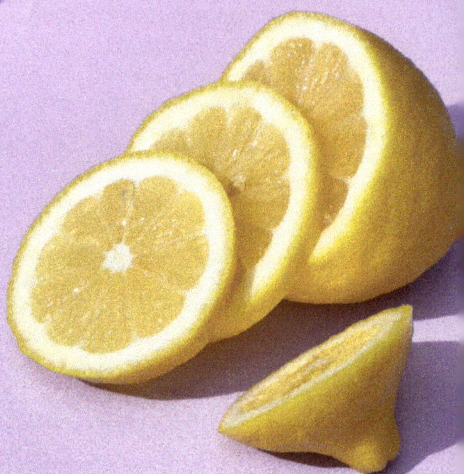

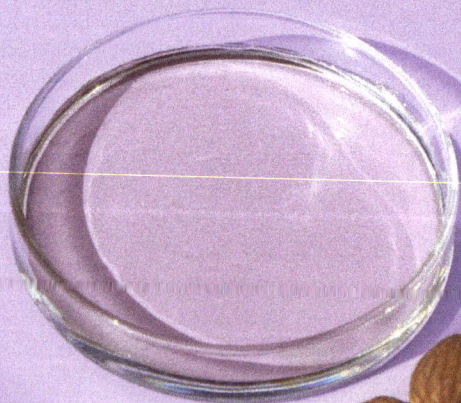

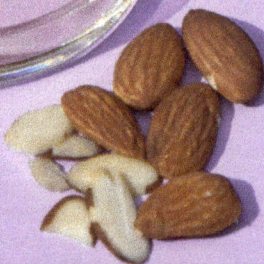

71. CHOCOLATE ANTI POLLUTION MASK

INGREDIENTS:

- 1/2 large spoon of cocoa powder.
- 3 squares of melted dark chocolate.
- 1 teaspoon of vegetable walnut oil, (almond / macadamia oil).
- 2 drops of vitamin E.
- 2 drops of fresh lemon.
- 2 large spoons of Greek yogurt.

DIRECTIONS:

- In 1 medium bowl, collect all the ingredients.
- Using a spatula, mix vigorously until you obtain a smooth / homogeneous cream.
- Using a brush, spread the mask over the face (avoid eye area) and neck.
- Keep the mask on for 20 minutes
- Rinse off the mask with lukewarm water.
- With a compress soaked in witch hazel water, wash off the rest of the mask. Massage the face with 2 drops of vitamin E oil.

72. BEAUTY AND FRESHNESS MASK (FOR ALL SKIN TYPES)

INGREDIENTS: TYPES-10 DROPS OF ORGANIC TAMANU OIL.

- 2 drops of lavender essential oil.
- 1/4 of fresh lemon juice.
- 2 large spoons of sour cream.
- 1 egg yolk.
- 1 teaspoon of honey.
- 1/2 spoon of avocado.

DIRECTIONS:

- In a small bowl, combine all the ingredients.
- Using a spatula, mix well until a smooth cream is obtained. with a brush, spread the mask over the face and neck. keep the mask on for 15 to 20 minutes.
- Rinse off with lukewarm water.
- Using a compress soaked in Aloe Vera water, wash off the rest of the mask.
- Finish with a moisturizer.

73. BANANA MASK (FOR OILY SKIN)

INGREDIENTS:

- 3 large spoons of Greek yogurt.
- 3 drops of grapefruit essential oil.
- 2 teaspoons of organic rose water.
- 1 large spoon of Aloe Vera gel.
- 1/2 mashed banana.

DIRECTIONS:

- In 1 medium bowl, pour all the ingredients.
- Using a spatula, mix well until a smooth cream is obtained.
- Using a brush, spread the mask over the face and neck, avoiding the eye area.
- Keep the mask on for 25 to 30 minutes.
- Rinse with lukewarm water. Soak a compress in Aloe Vera water, cleanse the skin well. Finish with a moisturizer.

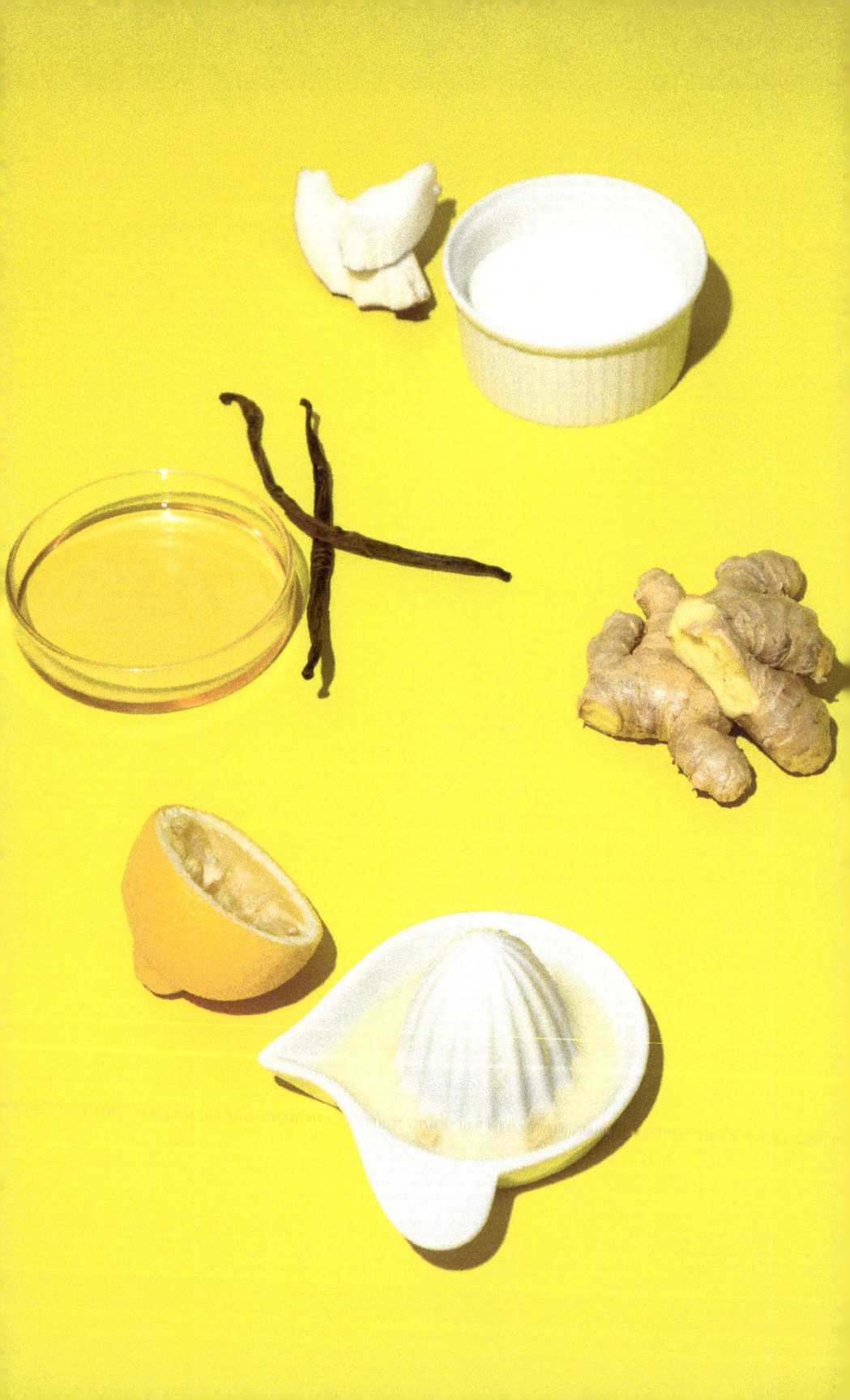

74. FACE SCRUB— UNIFIED COMPLEXION

MATERIAL:

- 1 medium bowl.
- 1 spatula.

INGREDIENTS:

- 1/2 squeezed lemon juice.
- 1 teaspoon of vanilla.
- 1/2 cup of warm organic coconut milk.
- 5 drops of liquid organic silicon.
- 1/4 teaspoon of organic ginger powder.
- 1 pinch of powder of vitamin C.
- 2 drops of vitamin E.

INSTRUCTIONS FOR USE:

- Pour the ginger powder and the powder of vitamin C.
- Add the warm coconut milk to the bowl. Using the spatula, mix well the ingredients for 1 minute to obtain a dough without lumps. add the remaining ingredients to the bowl.
- Using the spatula, continue to mix for 2 minutes.
- Let cool, then spread this peeling scrub on the face, avoiding the eye area. Keep the peeling scrub for 10-13 minutes.
- Using your fingertips, perform a circular massage for 2 minutes.
- Rinse off with lukewarm water. dry your skin and use 1 cream based on collagen and vitamin A.

Oils and Body Milk

75. AVOCADO BODY CREAM

MATERIAL:

- 1 wooden fork.
- 1 small saucepan.
- 1 deep plate.
- 1 small blender.
- 1 wooden spatula.
- 1 empty cream jar of 100ml.

INGREDIENTS:

- 1 small ripe avocado.
- 6 spoons of organic Shea butter.
- 4 large spoons of macadamia oil / organic linseed oil.
- 2 drops of vitamin E / 4 drops of Cosgard preservative.
- 5 drops of rose / cornflower essential oil.
- 15 drops of floral water / hydrosol of your choice.

DIRECTIONS:

- Using a wooden fork, crush half of the avocado flesh. pour the flesh of the crushed half avocado into the small saucepan, add 6 spoons of shea butter and 4 large spoons of macadamia oil to the saucepan.
- Turn on the heat, and put the pan on low heat, using the wooden spatula, mix all these ingredients well until the avocado and shea butter have completely melted.
- Take the pan out of the heat and continue to mix for 3 minutes.
- Pour the contents of the saucepan into 1 deep plate / large bowl.

- Add the 2nd half of the avocado flesh as well as the essential oils and the rest of the ingredients, including the floral water.
- Using the small blender, mix all the ingredients to obtain 1 fluid and smooth cream.
- Pour this cream into the bottle, close the bottle and place it in the refrigerator for 20 minutes.
- Use this body cream after each bath / shower.

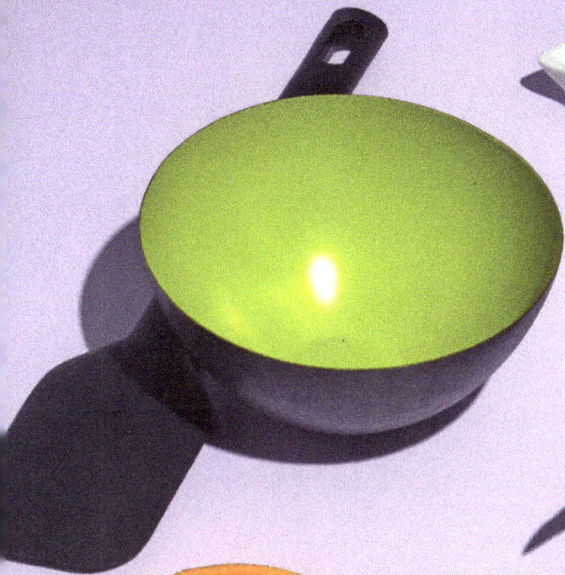

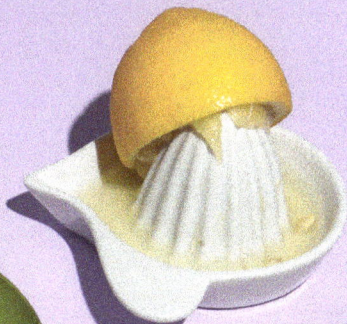

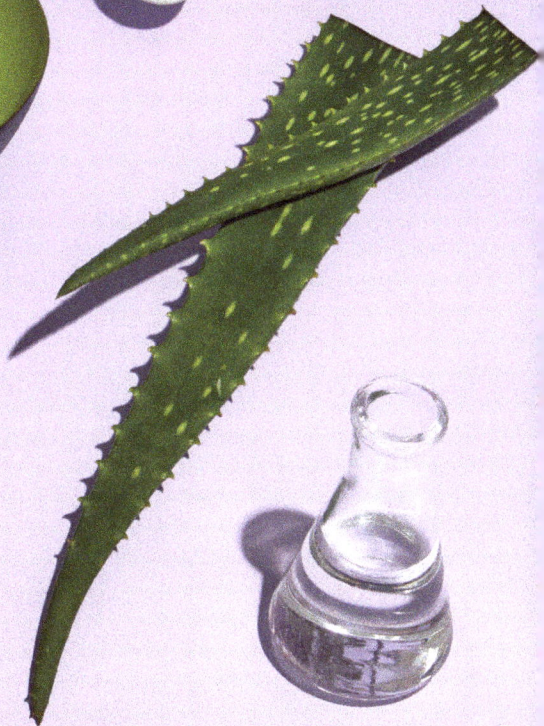

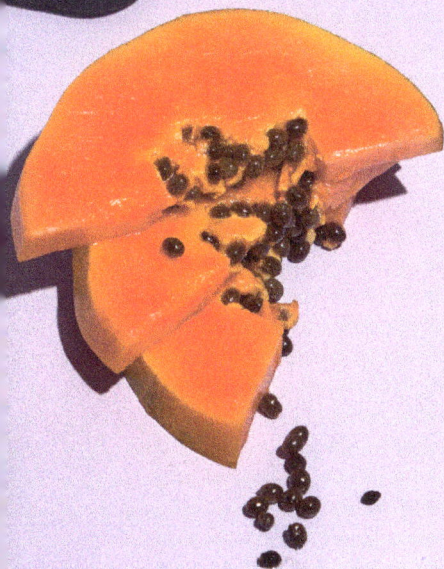

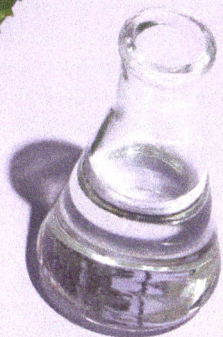

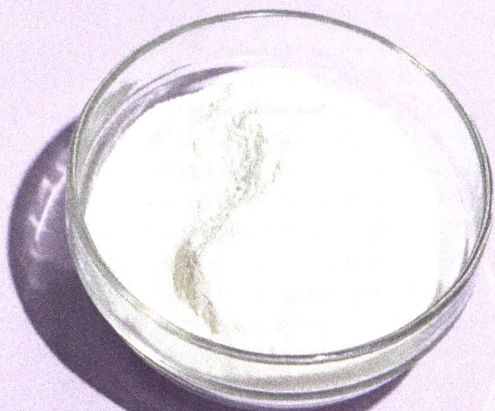

76. PEELING BODY SCRUB WITH PAPAYA FRUIT POWDER

MATERIAL:

- 1 small bowl.
- 1 spatula.

INGREDIENTS:

- 3 large spoons of rice flour.
- 1 teaspoon of papaya fruit powder.
- 1 large spoon of organic Aloe Vera gel.
- 1 juice of 1 fresh squeezed lemon.
- 1 teaspoon of glycerin.

INSTRUCTIONS FOR USE:

- Pour all the ingredients into the small bowl.
- Using the spatula, mix the ingredients well until obtained smooth paste.
- Spread this peeling scrub on the body. Perform a local circular massage for 5 minutes.
- Rinse off with lukewarm water. Pat your skin dry, then use a moisturizing lotion body.

77. ANTI-CELLULITE LOTION WITH COFFEE AND AVOCADO

MATERIAL:

- 1 PET bottle of 100 ml.
- 1 coffee filter.
- 1 horsehair glove.

INGREDIENTS:

- 2 large spoons of ground black coffee.
- 1 large cup of 100 ml of hot water.
- 1 large spoon of organic avocado vegetable oil.
- 4 drops of essential oil of ginger.
- 4 drops of eucalyptus essential oil.

INSTRUCTIONS FOR USE:

- In the coffee machine, pour 1 large cup of water and filter the ground coffee.
- Once the filtered coffee, pour it into the 100ml glass.
- Let the coffee cool. Then pour the coffee into the bottle.
- Add organic avocado oil and essential oils to the bottle.
- Close the bottle tightly. Shake it for 1 minute.
- Shake the bottle well before each use.
- On the horsehair glove, pour a few drops of this preparation and vigorously massage the areas with cellulite for 3 minutes.
- Keep this oil on your skin for 5 hours.
- Take your shower, dry your skin.
- Repeat this anti cellulite treatment 3 times / week.

78. NOURISHING AFTER SHOWER CREAM FOR THE BODY

MATERIAL:

- 1 medium bowl.
- 1 spatula.
- 1 empty 60 ml jar of cream.
- 1 mini mixer / mini mixer.

INGREDIENTS :

- 30 ml of organic hazelnut vegetable oil.
- 25 ml of linseed / grape seed oil.
- 3 large spoons of beeswax / coconut butter.
- 4 large spoons of orange / cornflower floral water.
- 1 teaspoon of glycerin oil there.

DIRECTIONS:

- In the bowl, pour the vegetable oils, beeswax / coconut butter.
- Place the bowl in the Marie bath.
- Using the spatula, mix all these ingredients well for 1 minute.
- Remove the bowl from the bain-marie. Using the mini blender, blend for 1 minute.
- add the hydrosol / floral water to the bowl.
- Add the essential oils and continue mixing with the blender for a period of 2 minutes, until you obtain a smooth and firm cream.
- Pour this cream into the pot. Close the jar. you can store this cream in a cool and ventilated place.

79. ESSENTIAL SHOWER GEL

INGREDIENTS:

- OIL-Purchase 1 bottle with neutral unscented shower gel.
- 5 drops of grapefruit essential oil.
- 4 drops of small grain essential oil.
- 6 drops of rosemary essential oil.
- 1 soft horsehair glove.

DIRECTIONS:

- Add all the essential ingredients to the bottle.
- Close the bottle tightly.
- Before taking each shower, shake the bottle vigorously,
- Use this shower gel in synergy with the horsehair glove. Insist on the cellulite parts. Keep the gel 2 minutes before rinsing.

80. ANTI ODOR BALM FOR FEET RECIPE

MATERIAL:

- 2 medium bowls.
- 1 spatula.
- 1 empty cream jar of 50 ml.
- 1 mini blender.

INGREDIENTS:

- 5 large spoons of argan vegetable oil / organic borage oil.
- 2 large spoons of avocado vegetable oil / Shea oil.
- 3 large spoons of beeswax.
- 2 large spoons of bicarbonate powder.
- 1 large spoon of grape seed oil.
- 3 drops of grapefruit essential oil.
- 3 drops of essential oil of ginger
- 2 drops of essential oil of tea tree.
- 1 large spoonful of zinc oxide powder.
- 1 large spoonful of white clay powder.
- 1 large spoon of potato starch powder.

DIRECTIONS:

- In 1 bowl, mix the potato starch, oxide zinc powder and white clay powder.
- Add the essential oils. using the spatula, mix all the ingredients well until obtained a smooth paste is.
- In the 2nd bowl, pour beeswax and vegetable oils.
- Place the bowl in the bain-marie, continue to mix the ingredients using the spatula.

∽ Remove the bowl from the bain-marie, then mix in the bowl, using a mixer for a period of 1 minute to obtain a smooth paste.

∽ Gather the contents of the ingredients of the 2 bowls in the pot.

∽ Before each use of this balm, have your feet, dry them, then massage your feet with this balm, insisting between the toes.

∽ Repeat this twice a week.

81. ANTI-CAPITON SLIMMING SEAWEED GEL

MATERIAL:

- 1 PET bottle of 100 ml.

INGREDIENTS:

- 60 ml of organic Aloe Vera gel.
- 20 ml of organic spirulina algae gel extract.
- 10 ml of Nigella / jojoba vegetable oil.
- 5 ml of floral water / chamomile hydrosol.
- 25 drops of Ravensara essential oil.
- 10 drops of essential oil of ginger.
- 10 drops of mandarin essential oil.

INSTRUCTIONS FOR USE:

- Pour all the ingredients into the bottle.
- Close the bottle tightly, shake the bottle for 2 minutes.
- Use this oil in a local massage on the parts with cellulite.

82. ANTI-CELLULITE PLANT CREAM

MATERIAL:

- 1 bottle of 100 ml in PET.

INGREDIENTS:

- 25 ml of evening primrose / sesame vegetable oil.
- 10 ml of sunflower vegetable oil.
- 2 large spoons of organic Aloe Vera gel.
- 60 ml of floral water / rosemary hydrosol.
- 2 large spoons of active caffeine powder.
- 5 drops of rosemary essential oil.
- 5 drops of Ravensara essential oil.

INSTRUCTIONS FOR USE:

- Pour all the ingredients into the bottle.
- Close the bottle tightly, shake it for 3 minutes.
- Shake the bottle well before each use. with this oil, massage the cellulite parts for 5 minutes.

83. NOURISHING STRAWBERRY BODY BALM

MATERIALS:

- 1 blender.
- 1 wooden spatula.
- 1 glass jar of 60 ml.

INGREDIENTS:

- 50 g of fresh strawberries.
- 5 ml of vegetable oil of hazelnuts.
- 1/2 fresh squeezed lemon juice.
- 2 drops of zinc.
- 1/2 teaspoon of ginger extract powder.
- 5 drops of glycerin.
- 2 drops of vitamin E.

INSTRUCTIONS FOR USE:

- Pour all the ingredients into the blender.
- Blend for 2 minutes.
- Pour this cream into the cream jar. keep this cream in the refrigerator for up to 2 weeks.

84. SLIMMING BODY CREAM WITH AVOCADO

MATERIAL:

- 1 medium bowl.
- 1 flat plate.
- 1 fork.
- 1 spatula.

INGREDIENTS:

- 1 small fresh avocado.
- 4 drops of verbena essential oil.
- 3 drops of essential oil from my fat.
- Juice of 1 fresh squeezed lemon.
- 1 large spoon of acacia honey.
- 1/4 teaspoon of vitamin C powder.
- 1/4 teaspoon of brown seaweed powder.
- 1/2 teaspoon of Vegetable collagen gel.
- 4 drops of glycerin.

INSTRUCTIONS FOR USE:

- Cut the avocado in 2. Collect the avocado pulp.
- In the flat plate, mash the avocado with the fork.
- Pour the avocado pulp into the bowl.
- Add all the ingredients to the bowl. Using the spatula, mix all the ingredients together to obtain a smooth and homogeneous paste.
- Massage the cellulite areas for 5 minutes with this cream.
- Repeat this anti cellulite treatment 3 times / week.

85. SLIMMING GELLING PLANT CREAM

MATERIAL:

- 1 glass jar of 250 ml.
- 1 spatula.
- 1 large bowl.

INGREDIENTS:

- 2 teaspoons of matcha powder.
- 6 drops of organic geranium essential oil.
- 6 drops of grapefruit essential oil.
- 1 large spoon of organic glycerin.
- 200 ml of floral water / mineral water.
- 1/2 teaspoon of liquid rice protein.
- 1/2 teaspoon of vegetable charcoal powder.
- 2 small spoons of organic Aloe Vera gel.

DIRECTIONS:

- Pour all the ingredients into the large bowl.
- Using the spatula, mix the ingredients well for 3 minutes until a smooth and homogeneous paste is obtained.
- Pour this paste into the bottle. Close the bottle.
- Use this paste in a local massage on the parts with cellulite.
- Keep on the skin for 2 hours, rinse with lukewarm water.
- Repeat this treatment 3 times / week.

86. VELVETY MOISTURIZING CREAM FOR THE BODY

MATERIAL:

- 1 small saucepan.
- 1 large bowl. hand mixer / whisk.
- 1 wooden spatula.
- 1 empty glass jar of 100 ml.

INGREDIENTS:

- 1 large slice of Shea butter.
- 30 ml of rose water / other hydrosol of your choice.
- 20 ml of organic aloe Vera gel.
- 5 drops of vitamin E.
- 10 drops of essential oil of cypress.
- 50 ml of organic coconut vegetable oil.
- 15 drops of rose essential oil.

INSTRUCTIONS FOR USE:

- Pour the slice of shea butter into the small saucepan.
- Place the pan on low heat.
- Once the shea butter has melted, remove the pan from the heat.
- Let cool. Pour the melted shea butter into the bowl. add all the ingredients to the bowl.
- Mix well for 3 minutes.
- Place the bowl in the refrigerator for 10 minutes. Take the bowl out of the refrigerator.
- Using the wooden spatula, continue mixing for 1 minute.
- Pour the cream into the pot.
- Store this cream in a cool place.

87. LEMON BODY CREAM

MATERIAL:

- 1 large bowl.
- 1 mixer / mixer.
- 1 spatula.
- 1 empty glass jar of 350 ml.

INGREDIENTS:

- 100 g of coconut / shea butter.
- 100 g of organic carrot vegetable oil.
- 100g of mango butter / Aloe Vera gel.
- 50 g of glycerin.
- 4 small teaspoons of beeswax.
- 1 fresh squeezed lemon juice.
- 3 drops of Cosgard preservative / 3 drops of vitamin E.

INSTRUCTIONS FOR USE:

- In the large bowl, pour the shea butter and beeswax.
- Place the bowl in a bain-marie, with the spatula mix the ingredients until the beeswax and shea butter melt.
- Remove the bowl from the bain-marie.
- Add the vegetable carrot oil to the bowl, continue mixing the ingredients in the bowl.
- Place the bowl in the refrigerator for 1h30.
- Take the bowl out of the fridge, add the lemon juice and the rest of the essential oils. Continue to mix well until you obtain a homogeneous and smooth cream. Pour the cream into the jar. Close the jar. And keep this cream in the fridge.
- Use this body cream 3 times / week.

88. BODY OIL WITH ESSENTIAL OILS AFTER SHOWER

MATERIAL:

- 1 glass bottle of 100 ml with pipette.

INGREDIENTS:

- 40 g of melted Shea butter / coconut butter.
- 30g of organic Aloe Vera gel.
- 15 drops of carrot essential oil.
- 15 drops of liquid organic silicon.
- 10 drops of allantoin active
- 10 drops of liquid rice protein.
- 5 drops of vitamin E.

INSTRUCTIONS FOR USE:

- In the bottle, combine all interference.
- Close the bottle, shake for 2 minutes.
- Use this regenerating body oil after each shower.

89. ANTI STRETCH MARK BODY OIL

MATERIAL:

- 1 glass bottle of 30 ml

INGREDIENTS:

- 25 ml of organic hazelnut vegetable oil.
- 1 teaspoon of organic carrot oil.
- 3 drops of lavender essential oil.
- 4 drops of mandarin essential oil.

INSTRUCTIONS FOR USE:

- Pour all the ingredients into the glass bottle.
- Close the bottle tightly. Shake well for 1 minute.
- Every evening uses a few drops of this oil in a local massage on the stretch marks.
- This recipe is also suitable for post pregnancy.

90. CIRCULATORY TONING LEG OIL AND ANTI OEDEMAS

MATERIAL:

- 1 glass bottle of 30ml.

INGREDIENTS:

- 25 ml of organic wheat germ vegetable oil / almond oil.
- 6 drops of geranium sentinel oil.
- 10 drops of essential oil of Cypress.

INSTRUCTIONS FOR USE:

- Pour all the ingredients into the bottle.
- Close the bottle tightly, shake it for 1 minute.
- In the evening, use a few drops of this oil and massage your legs from the ankle upwards until the oil is completely absorbed into the skin.
- Do not rinse. Keep this oil on the skin overnight.

91. BODY SCRUB WITH COCONUT AND BROWN SUGAR

INGREDIENTS:

- 50 g / 3 large spoons of coconut vegetable oil.
- 60 g / 3 large spoons of brown sugar powder.
- 10 drops of lavender / lemon essential oil.
- 4 drops of vitamin E.

DIRECTIONS:

- Pour vegetable coconut oil in 1 medium bowl.
- Place the bowl in the Marie bath, mix well until the sugar in the oil melts.
- Add the essential oils and vitamin E.
- Remove the bowl from the bain-marie, mix the ingredients well with a spatula.
- Pour this lotion into the bottle / jar.
- Let cool.
- Before the shower, use this scrub on your body.
- Using a soft horsehair glove, massage your body.
- Rinse your scrub well in the shower.
- Use this body peel 3X / week.

92. JOJOBA AND LEMON BODY BALM ANTI STRETCH MARKS

INGREDIENTS:

- 1 bottle / 100 ml glass jar.
- 6 drops of vitamin E.
- 1 teaspoon of glycerin.
- 15 ml of argan / macadamia oil.
- 20 ml of avocado vegetable oil.
- 30 ml of linseed oil / jojoba oil.
- 20 ml of shea oil / sunflower oil.
- 10 drops of lemon / rose essential oil.

DIRECTIONS:

- Pour all ingredients into 1 medium bowl.
- Place the bowl in the Marie bath. Mix well with 1 spatula.
- Let cool . Pour the balm into the bottle / jar.
- Mass the parts of the body with this balm, keep it a few hours before showering. You can keep it on the skin for several hours / 1 night.

93. BODY RECIPE WITH LAVENDER, ANTI STRETCH MARKS

- 1 glass bottle of 30 ml.
- 25 ml of sweet almond oil.
- 1 small spoonful of seed oil (Seat) / organic hemp oil.
- 4 drops of lavender essential oil.
- 6 drops of mandarin essential oil.

DIRECTIONS:

- Gather all the ingredients in the glass bottle.
- Close the bottle tightly. Shake the bottle vigorously
- (for a period of one minute).
- Mass with this oil the parts of stretch marks.
- This recipe is also suitable for post pregnancy.
- Use this formula in local massage, every day.

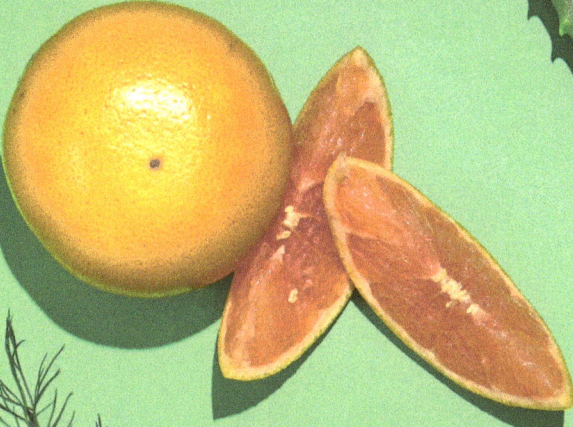

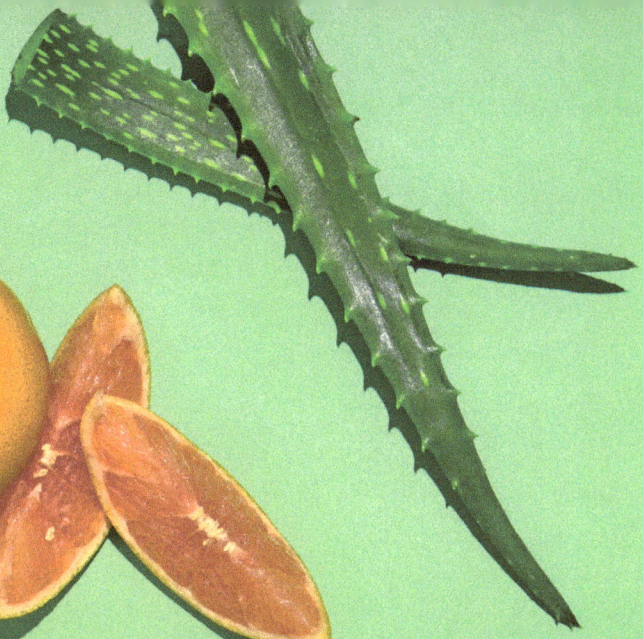

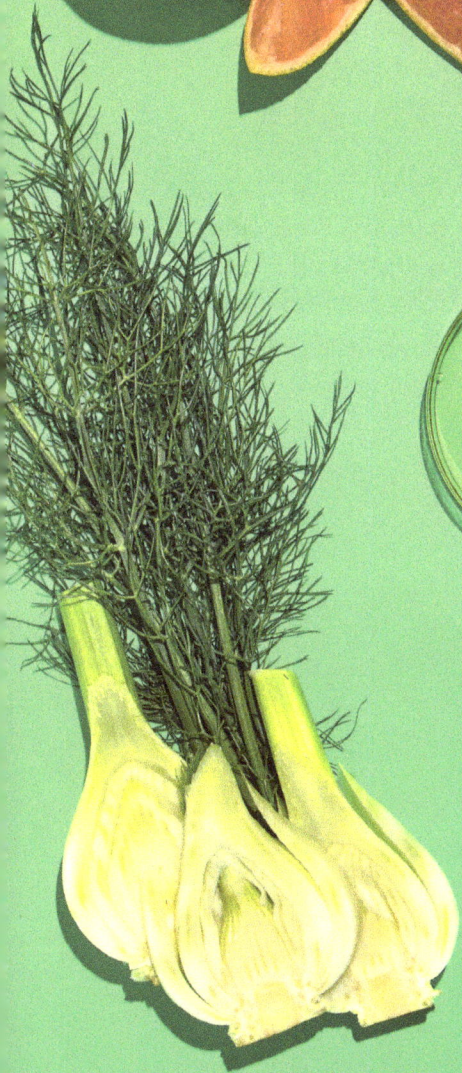

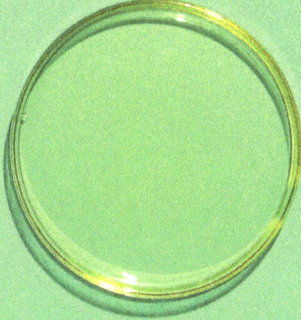

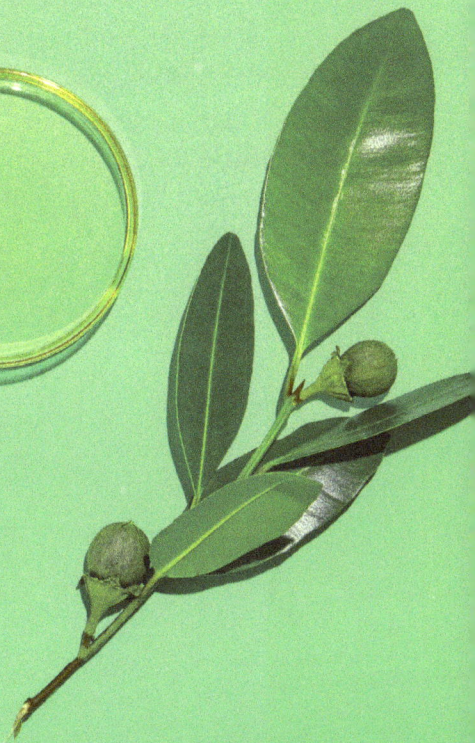

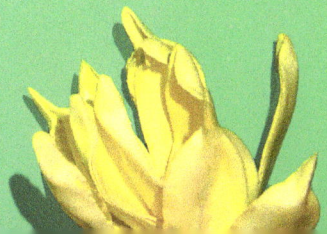

94. FENNEL DRAINING MASSAGE OIL

INGREDIENTS:

- 1 glass bottle of 30ml.
- 30 ml of organic jojoba vegetable oil.
- 6 drops of fennel vegetable oil.
- 15 drops of grapefruit essential oil.

INSTRUCTIONS FOR USE:

- Pour all the ingredients into the bottle.
- Close the bottle and shake the bottle for 2 minutes. every evening, after your bath for 5 minutes. massage with this oil the parts where cellulite appears.
- Keep on the skin overnight.

Men's Recipes

95. NATURAL PLANT BEARD OIL

MATERIAL:

- 1 bowl.
- 1 spatula / small whisk.
- 1 empty syringe of 10ml.
- 1 bottle with 40 ml glass / PET pump.

INGREDIENTS:

- 10 ml of borage / macadamia vegetable oil.
- 10 ml of linseed / coconut vegetable oil.
- 13 ml of organic argan / castor vegetable oil.
- 2 drops of frankincense essential oil.

DIRECTIONS:

- Gather all the ingredients in the bowl.
- Mix the ingredients well for 2 minutes.
- Transfer your ready oil into the bottle.
- Use this oil 1-2 times a day while straightening your beard.

96. LEMON LAVENDER SPRAY DEODORANT

MATERIAL:

- 1 bowl.
- 1 spatula / 1 mini whisk.
- 1 small ladle of 100 ml.
- 1 pump bottle with glass / PET spray.

INGREDIENTS:

- 30 ml of Aloe Vera organic water / mineral water.
- 4 1/2 teaspoons (5g) of alum stone powder.
- 60 ml of witch hazel / mint hydrosol.
- 5 drops of lemon essential oil.
- 3 drops of organic lavender essential oil.

DIRECTIONS:

- Gather all the ingredients in the bowl.
- With the spatula / mini whisk, mix all the ingredients well for 2 minutes.
- Transfer your deodorant to the bottle.
- Close your bottle tightly and shake your bottle well before each use.

97. PURIFYING MEN'S TONIC WITH BAMBOO AND ESSENTIAL OILS

MATERIAL:

- 1 glass spray bottle of 50 ml.
- 1 sterile plastic syringe of 50 ml.
- 15 ml of lime blossom or witch hazel hydrosol.
- 12 ml of BAMBOO hydrosol.
- 10 ml of jasmine water / verbena hydrosol.
- 10 ml of orange blossom water.
- 10 drops of YLANG YLANG essential oil.
- 5 drops of hyaluronic acid or 4 drops of vitamin E.

INSTRUCTIONS FOR USE:

- Using the funnel, pour all the ingredients into the bottle.
- Close the bottle. Shake vigorously for 2 minutes.
- Use this tonic spray on the face 3 times / week (avoid eye area).

98. CALENDULA POST SHAVE CALMING GEL FOR MEN

MATERIAL:

- 1 glass / PET bottle of 100 ml.

INGREDIENTS:

- 15 ml of organic hemp oil.
- 55 ml of organic Aloe Vera gel.
- 20 ml of organic calendula oil.
- 30 drops of organic Tamanu oil.
- 10 ml of organic hazelnut vegetable oil.

INSTRUCTIONS FOR USE:

- Pour all the ingredients into the bottle.
- Close the bottle tightly. Shake it
- For 1 minute store the bottle in 1 dry and cool place.
- After each sun exposure, apply a few drops of this gel to the skin.

99. AFTER SHAVE GINGER MOISTURIZING GEL

MATERIAL:

- 1 medium bowl.
- 1 pipette bottle of 50 ml.
- 1 empty sterile syringe of 2 ml.
- 1 spatula / or mini whisk.

INGREDIENTS:

- 3 drops of essential oil of ginger.
- 10 drops of organic cornflower / helichrysum essential oil.
- 5 drops of organic lavender essential oil.
- 45 ml of organic Aloe Vera gel.
- 3 ml of linseed / avocado vegetable oil.
- 3 drops of organic tamanu oil.
- 3 drops of cosgard preservative / 3 drops of vitamin E.

INSTRUCTIONS FOR USE:

- Pour all the ingredients into the bowl.
- Using the spatula / mini whisk, mix all the ingredients for 1 minute.
- Using the syringe, pour the gel into the vial.
- Place the cap on the quilts, close the bottle with its cap.
- Shake the bottle well before each use.
- Use this gel after each shave.

100. MOISTURIZING AND SOFTENING AFTER SHAVE CREAM

INGREDIENTS:

- 1 medium bowl.
- 1 bottle with a pipette / jar of 50ml.
- 40 ml of peppermint / chamomile hydrosol.
- 1/2 teaspoon of organic glycerin.
- 1/2 teaspoon of organic ginger powder.
- 20 drops of organic linseed / macadamia oil.
- 1/2 teaspoon of organic aloe vera gel.
- 1/2 teaspoon of vitamin C / or almond milk powder.

DIRECTIONS:

- In the bowl, pour the ginger powder and the almond milk powder.
- Add the peppermint / chamomile hydrosol.
- Mix the ingredients well.
- Add glycerin, linseed / macadamia oil and continue mixing until you obtain a smooth cream.
- Add the rest of the ingredients and continue to mix for 1 minute.
- Pour the cream into the bottle / jar and keep the jar of cream in a cool place.

MY BEAUTY PRODUCTS WEBSITE:

WWW.CAMILLEOBADIA.COM

TO RECEIVE 15% DISCOUNT ON PRODUCTS USE CODE "CAMILLEBOOK" DURING CHECKOUT

MY BEAUTY CLINIC WEBSITE:

WWW.BEAUTEOBLIGE.COM

www.ingramcontent.com/pod-product-compliance
Lightning Source LLC
Chambersburg PA
CBHW052112030426
42335CB00025B/2953